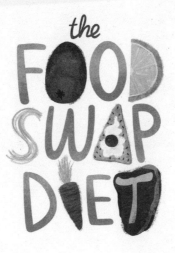

Discover the food swaps that will transform
your diet and your weight – permanently

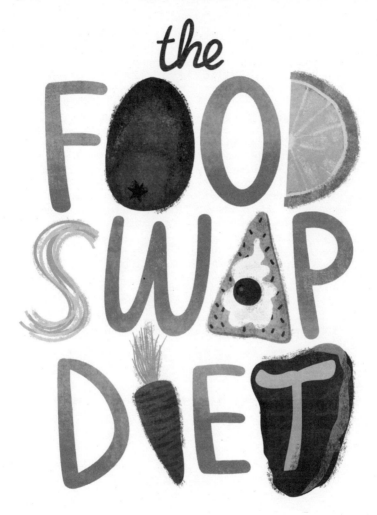

the FOOD SWAP DIET

PETA BEE

piatkus

PIATKUS

First published in Great Britain in 2013 by Piatkus
Reprinted 2013

A CIP catalogue record for this book
is available from the British Library.

ISBN 978-0-7499-5783-4

Design and typesetting by Paul Saunders
Printed and bound in Great Britain by Clays Ltd, St Ives plc

Papers used by Piatkus are from well-managed forests
and other responsible sources.

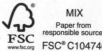

MIX
Paper from
responsible sources
FSC
www.fsc.org   FSC® C104740

PIATKUS
An imprint of
Little, Brown Book Group
100 Victoria Embankment
London EC4Y 0DY

Peta Bee is an award-winning journalist with degrees in sports science and nutrition. She writes articles on health and fitness in *The Times* and contributes to the *Sunday Times* and *Daily Mail* as well as being contributing editor of *Women's Running* magazine. Peta has appeared widely on television and radio and is the author of five previous books including *The Official 2012 London Olympics Fitness Guide for Women* (Carlton). She is a former winner of Fitness Professional of the Year and she won the Medical Journalists' Association's Freelancer of the Year award in 2008 and 2012.

Contents

Acknowledgements

THANK YOU, FIRST OF ALL, TO THE many people who have shared their concerns about particular foods and ingredients with me. Unwittingly, you have provided the basis of this book.

Thank you to my agent, Robert Smith, for his encouragement and belief in the idea, to Anne Lawrence, of Piatkus, Little, Brown, for taking the project on, and to Jillian Stewart and Jan Cutler for their guidance and patience.

There are many experts who have helped me to decipher jargon and navigate the food industry maze, in particular the dieticians of the British Dietetic Association, the nutrition scientists of the British Nutrition Foundation and the experts at the Institute of Food Research and the MRC Human Nutrition Research centre. Thanks to them and to anyone else who has been plagued by my emails and phone calls.

Finally, a big thank you to the food manufacturers and retailers that willingly provide easy-to-read lists of ingredients and nutritional profiles for their products (but no thanks to those who don't).

Introduction

THERE WAS NO SINGLE REASON why I began to 'food swap', no eureka moment that prompted me to immediately re-evaluate what I was eating and feeding my family. In retrospect, it was probably a gradual gnawing away at my conscience, a realisation that the food we eat has become over-complicated to the point of mass confusion, that led to this book. There are many occasions when I can recall food discussions with other mothers at the school gates that had triggered alarm bells to ring in my head. Or times when I have heard or read about food industry or dietary absurdities that have left me bewildered.

My overriding hunch has always been that eating for good health should be simple and straightforward, that we can all achieve good nutritional habits if only we can learn to navigate the minefield that our food supply has become. That became the underlying principle of *The Food Swap Diet*. In the course of my research for the pages that follow, I have scrutinised nutritional profiles of hundreds of foods, consulted leading experts and hopefully unravelled some of the mysteries surrounding the products we put into our shopping trolleys every week. The result is that within each chapter there are numerous suggested food swaps or choices that will help to cut calories, fat and sugar from your diet by replacing a less than favourable food with a nutritionally superior choice.

We live in a world where sugary cereals laced with synthetic vitamins contribute towards a significant chunk of our nutrient intake, where desserts are high in salt, pizzas are loaded with sugar and where a sweetened can of baked beans can count as a vegetable. As the choice of foods available to us have expanded beyond expectation, so too have the lists of scientific-sounding ingredients designed to trick our palates into craving more of them. So confusing has it become that we can be forgiven for not knowing what we are putting into our mouths on a daily basis.

Foods we buy because they look wholesome can be loaded with unimaginably high levels of fat, sugar, salt or additives. Many of the labels we faithfully assume to be providing us with accurate information are at best misleading, at worst inaccurate. All too often, what we eat because we think it is good for us is anything but. Did you know, for example, that the wholesome-looking yoghurt dessert you pick up at lunchtime could contain more fat and calories than a quarterpounder burger? Or that a coffee drink that appears to be low fat might be more calorific than a bowl of trifle topped with fresh cream? A bag of ready-salted crisps probably contains far less salt than your sandwich, and your high-bran breakfast cereal more sugar than a chocolate bar. Even seemingly healthy salads can be a high-fat nightmare in disguise.

By becoming more aware of what you eat it is possible to achieve and maintain a healthy body without having to survive on rocket leaves. Losing weight is not just about keeping tabs on calories, fat and sugar; what I quickly discovered is that by swapping unhealthy options for wiser, more nutritious choices, metabolism can be boosted, hunger satiated and body fat reduced.

For me, food swapping has become a refreshingly straightforward way of life. I've become adept at comparing seemingly similar foods only to discover that one is far friendlier to the waistline than the other. I've uncovered the creative and, it has to be said, highly unnatural methods used by manufacturers to mislead and confuse our palates. I know what you should swap and what to drop in order to hit your weight-loss target. And I have come to realise that eating for health and slimness need not entail a torturous existence on mundane and limited foods.

How to use this book

The Food Swap Diet is intended to be as much a reference book as anything else – a manual into which you can dip for guidance when you need it. As such, each chapter can be digested as a stand-alone section with plenty of advice for changing your eating habits for the better. Where relevant, nutritional information is either per 'typical' product or the average values of the most widely available products of its kind.

In Chapter 1 I explain why my food swaps work compared to other diets and how they can fit successfully into a busy lifestyle. Chapter 2 delves into the murky world of labelling and steers you towards making healthier food with tips on how to read information on food packaging. I also explain what the different food groups mean and their importance in your overall diet along with how many calories to eat to ensure a steady and healthy weight loss.

Chapters 3 to 9 list the swaps and healthy choices you can make to fill your store-cupboard and fridge and to provide three meals a day as well as snacks and a coffee break. In Chapter 10, the focus is on what to feed your children without falling prey to marketing and labelling cons, and Chapter 11 helps you avoid the high-calorie pitfalls of eating out. Finally, Chapter 12 looks at the numerous drinks available and how you can choose selectivity to avoid adding extra unnecessary calories when trying to keep your fluids balanced.

My hope is that you will dip in and out of the sections as needed and become a proficient food swapper in your own right.

Food swapping is no flash-in-the-pan dietary fad. It is a long-term approach that works, something that won't lead to gnawing hunger pangs and frustrating binges. It can pave the way to more relaxed and enjoyable eating. And, most importantly, it can enhance your health and enable you to live life to the full, for longer. I hope the food swapping knowledge I have amassed through my research means this approach can enhance your life as it has done mine.

Peta Bee

CHAPTER **ONE**

Why food swaps work

THE CONCEPT OF FOOD SWAPPING is not new. For years, dieticians, nutritionists and government healthy-eating advisors have urged us to switch calorie-dense foods for those that are nutrient dense. But many of us have lost our way in the maze of dietary advice we face on a daily basis and no longer know how to choose and buy food to meet our nutritional requirements and the energy needs of our bodies. Day by day, it seems, we are offered different dietary advice. What is good for you one week is billed as an artery-clogger the next; a food that extends your life in one study is found to cut it short in another.

During the last 30 years, diets claiming to offer solutions to weight problems have come and gone. It's no coincidence, either, that this rise in fashionable diets has occurred during a time when healthy-eating guidelines centred on the now questionable advice to focus on low-fat and high-carbohydrate foods for weight loss. As you will discover later on, many low-fat foods are far from a healthy choice and are laced with sugar, additives

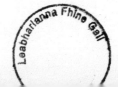

and salt instead. Combined with a corresponding slump in activity levels over the last three decades, the result is a level of obesity and weight problems worse than any in history.

While they differ in their delivery of the message, all successful diets have the same underlying formula as their premise: when you eat too much and move about too little, weight gain will occur. Studies suggest that calories really do matter in the battle of the bulge, including several published in the highly regarded *New England Journal of Medicine*. In one of those investigations, researchers put 811 overweight adults on one of four diets that differed according to their protein, fat and carbohydrate content. By the end of the study, everyone who cut 750 calories from their daily intake, regardless of which diet plan they followed, lost the same amount of weight. Reverse that scenario and the pounds will start to pile back on.

What type of food you eat also plays a hugely important part in determining the long-term success of a diet. Ultimately, though, the downfall of fashionable eating plans is that they are too restrictive, too limiting in the foods they allow and thus they require truck-loads of self-discipline to succeed.

A straightforward way to find success

Where *The Food Swap Diet* differs from other diets is in its free rein: no food is banned. You lose weight by making educated decisions and informed choices. What matters is that you make wiser and healthier choices each time you eat breakfast or lunch, a snack or a restaurant meal.

Use it regularly and you will learn to consume food that leaves you satiated so that you don't crave a sugar-burst when energy levels plummet. What's more, the food choices you make will have health benefits beyond improving your size and shape:

swap foods appropriately and your skin and hair will gleam, your body will become adept at warding off bugs and viruses and, in time, you will build resilience to a range of more serious illnesses and conditions that have the potential to kill.

The pages that follow are also packed with tips on how to survive the onslaught of food advertising and messages that contrive to convince you that because a food is labelled as healthy it merits inclusion in your diet. What you will discover is that many seemingly nutritious ready-made foods are anything but and are best avoided in favour of something natural and fresh. This book is designed to help you make straightforward and informed decisions about what you eat so that you will never need to starve, skip meals or fall into the hunger trap of yo-yo dieting again.

The healthy diet

What is a healthy diet? For years we have been fed the theory that the food we should eat to stay slim and healthy should be low in fat, particularly fats from animal sources such as dairy food, high in carbohydrates and as free as possible from additives and added sugar and salt. A better understanding of nutrition science has, in recent years, thrown some of these long-standing recommendations into question. While it is now accepted that certain dietary rules should be cast in stone – such as, eating a wholesome breakfast (see Chapter 5), staying well hydrated (see Chapter 12), consuming vitamins and minerals in sufficient amounts to support health and, wherever possible, preparing food fresh from natural sources – expert opinion has now shifted when it comes to some aspects of nutritional thinking.

Whereas we were once advised to consume a small ratio of protein to carbohydrate foods to avoid weight gain, research has now confirmed a shift in scientific consensus. What is now known is that not all carbohydrates are equal and that the fact they are often low in fat does not mean they will necessarily help you to lose weight. As you will discover later in this chapter, what matters is the *quality* of the carbohydrate eaten. Essentially this means you should consume less of the highly refined variety that sends blood sugar levels soaring (causing you to feel hungry again shortly after, and leading to weight gain) and more of the sustaining, wholegrain carbohydrates that have a more healthy effect on blood sugar levels.

Replacing white pasta and bread with wholemeal pasta and bread, and brown rice, and shifting the overall balance from carbohydrate to protein foods such as meat, poultry, fish, eggs, nuts and cheese is now considered by many to offer a long-term solution to weight problems.

It remains crucial not to cut out entire food groups (unless you need to for medical reasons), but the balance on your plate should be weighted towards healthy protein foods, plenty of vegetables and some good-quality carbs. As ever, the greater variety of foods you can consume, the better your chances are of maintaining a high intake of different nutrients. Skipping meals is not an option, but consuming better balanced foods will ensure you don't fall into the hunger and fatigue trap that is the curse of dieters.

HOW FOOD SWAPS MAKE A DIFFERENCE

Food swapping is an approach that suits all lifestyles, whether you are a busy mum who never has time to prepare meals for herself, a stressed-out office worker who

▶

eats on the run or someone who simply feels that they have been losing the battle of the bulge for way too long. In an ideal world, all food would be prepared fresh and from ingredients that are naturally sourced. In reality, many of us rely on more pre-packaged and ready-made foods than we would like. Where food swapping helps is in determining which of the deluge of products available offers the nutritionally superior option. Its biggest appeal is its simplicity, a factor that ensures you will be able to make positive changes that will last for life. Nothing could be more straightforward. Take a look at how it might impact on the typical daily calorie intake of an office worker or busy mum:

Office worker

SWAP ▸ Blueberry muffin (430 calories)
FOR ▸ Fruit scone (337 calories)

SWAP ▸ Medium latte (223 calories)
FOR ▸ Americano (8 calories)

SWAP ▸ Chicken Caesar and bacon wrap (617 calories)
FOR ▸ Chicken salad wrap (364 calories)

SWAP ▸ Chicken korma (820 calories)
FOR ▸ Chicken jalfrezi (420 calories)

SWAP ▸ Gin and tonic (213 calories)
FOR ▸ Pimm's and lemonade (85 calories)

Daily saving: 1,089 calories

▶

Busy mum

SWAP ▶ Pain au raisin (432 calories)
FOR ▶ 2 poached eggs on toast with grilled tomato
(249 calories)

SWAP ▶ Granola bar (397 calories)
FOR ▶ Palmine biscuit (75 calories)

SWAP ▶ Vanilla iced coffee (340 calories)
FOR ▶ Iced vanilla latte (255 calories)

SWAP ▶ Toasted club sandwich (534 calories)
FOR ▶ Cream cheese and smoked salmon bagel
(420 calories)

SWAP ▶ Chicken and bacon pasta bake (683 calories)
FOR ▶ Fish pie (399 calories)

Daily saving: 988 calories

Why exercise matters

For most people weight gain is a slow creep of 900g–1.3kg (2–3lb) a year – barely noticeable at first, but gradually enough to see you adjust your belt by several notches before, eventually, you need to go up a size in clothes. There is little doubt that inactivity compounds weight problems. Burn just 30 fewer calories a day by failing to raise yourself out of your chair often enough and you will gain 1.3kg (3lb) in 12 months without even eating more.

That doesn't necessarily mean you need to join a gym. What's missing from many of our lives is the sort of incidental activity that we used to take for granted. A lack of walking, household chores, pram-pushing, stair-climbing – indeed, just moving – is having a more profound effect on our waistlines and health than any failure to attend the gym. Indeed, one study found that people who took moderate amounts of this kind of daily activity burnt more calories overall than those who performed short but intense gym sessions at lunchtime or after work. After a tough workout, people typically limit their activity and either go back to their desk or relax for the evening, assuming that they have done enough. The message? Get moving – in any way you can.

Food swapping goes hand in hand with exercise, and the two can fit in easily with your lifestyle, but you also need to know how the food swaps work by understanding how to make healthier choices in the food you buy. I discuss this in the following chapter.

CHAPTER **TWO**

.

How to make healthier food choices

WITHIN THE PAGES OF this book are dozens of food swaps that slice calories and fat per serving, fill you up more or provide considerably more nutrients than a corresponding choice. As you become a proficient food swapper, you will find that you can interchange many of the swaps listed, avoiding the poor choices and substituting the better foods listed throughout the book.

In most cases you will find levels listed for calories, fat, sugars and salt in each food – more information on each of these important factors follows. Where one of these is not included, it is because that particular food type contains too little to be of relevance. As you will discover throughout the book, calories are not the only thing to check when it comes to losing or maintaining weight and improving your health.

There are Top Swap Tips dotted throughout each chapter. Use these to make sensible choices when you are shopping or cooking – see them as golden rules for successful food swapping in the long term. I've also included some general guidelines on how to buy foods such as vegetables and fruits that are generally healthy but which might have specifically different benefits. In such cases, one food is not necessarily better than another, it just offers different benefits, so direct swaps are not listed.

Getting to grips with food labelling

Descriptions of food on packaging can be highly misleading. A 'low-fat' food can be high in sugar; a 'reduced-sugar' food can be high in fat. Deciphering labelling terms is crucial for successful food swapping, so it's worth reading What the Descriptive Words on Packaging Mean (see page 40) before you get started.

Calories – how many do you need?

It is estimated that the average adult man with moderate activity levels has a daily requirement for 2,500 calories whereas a woman needs 2,000 to maintain weight and stay healthy. Those needs differ according to build, activity levels and age, but are a useful marker for most people. To lose weight, it is recommended that calorie consumption is reduced to 2,000 calories for men and 1,500 for women. The more active you are, however, the more calories you generally need in a day. It sounds straightforward, but with changes in food manufacturing processes and with misleading labelling, it is not uncommon to find that foods you presumed would be low in calories are in fact highly calorific.

Latest figures show that we consume 200 calories a day

more than we did three decades ago, an increase that corresponds with a decrease in activity levels and, unsurprisingly, a sharp rise in the number of people who are overweight or obese. Consuming 3,500 extra calories will eventually lay down 450g (1lb) of surplus body fat. That sounds like a lot of calories, but a coffee shop iced coffee or hot chocolate contains more than 500 calories. Drink one of those a day and in seven days you will have amassed enough calories to create 450g (1lb) of new body fat. That's 23.5kg (52 lb/3 stone 10lb) a year.

As you will discover as you start food swapping, calories are not all that matter when it comes to losing pounds or maintaining a healthy weight. The nutritional profile of a food – that is, the amount of fat, salt and sugar it contains, as well as the levels of vitamins and minerals – play a crucial role in determining how quickly it settles as body fat and how easily it satiates us before the next meal.

Carbohydrate – for energy

For years it was thought that eating mostly carbohydrates was the key to successful weight loss; increasingly today though, some forms of carbohydrate are seen as the enemy. On the side of the good guys are the slow-release carbohydrates like wholemeal bread, wholegrain pasta and brown rice that provide us with the nutrients we need for a healthy body, giving us energy and keeping us feeling full. They cause a very slight rise in our blood sugar level, which helps to improve our mood over a period of time, because it affects hormone levels in our brains slowly, keeping us content. Wholegrain foods contain the grain in its unrefined form, and they take an incredible amount of time to digest, generally keeping us fuller for longer. Foods like beans, sweet potatoes and pulses have a similar effect. These so-called complex carbohydrates have a low glycaemic index or GI (see pages 16–18) and are generally the variety used by athletes to provide a sustained energy release. They are perfect for keeping you going throughout the day.

The problem with refined carbs

Our collective consumption of simple, sugary carbohydrates, such as white bread, white pasta and rice, as well as cakes, biscuits and sugary drinks, is now so high that they are considered a prime reason why so many people are overweight. Although the war against refined, sugary foods is in its relative infancy, it is likely to become a focus for government health and nutrition advisors the world over in the next decade. Already, bold moves are being made against sugary carbs. In New York in 2012, the mayor announced plans to ban supersized fizzy drinks in quantities of more than 600ml (20fl oz/1 pint) after the city's health commissioner linked New York's highest obesity rates to areas where the most sugary drinks were consumed.

What happens when too many refined carbohydrates are consumed is that blood sugar (glucose) rises sharply and the pancreas pumps out insulin ferociously to extract glucose from the bloodstream, convert it to glycogen and store it in the liver or muscles. Consume too high a carbohydrate content for too long, however, and this process is compromised. About an hour and a half after eating refined carbs you feel hungry again, so you eat more and the result is that since the body has a limited capacity for glycogen storage, excess is stored as body fat. Eventually, overloaded by the sugary demands, the body becomes 'insulin resistant' and this paves the way for type-2 diabetes. Since insulin is the main hormone responsible for depositing fat cells, many obesity experts now propose that a lower and healthier carbohydrate diet will reduce insulin levels and release stored body fat for use as fuel.

Spikes in blood sugar levels from eating too many sugary carbs are now linked to a host of other unhealthy side effects. They are known to be linked to the action of the hormone leptin, secreted by fat cells to act on a part of the brain that suppresses appetite and controls metabolism. When someone gains weight, leptin levels rise in a bid to maintain the equilibrium. But huge swings in blood sugar can lead to 'leptin resistance', meaning the hormone is unable to do its job and the body settles at a weight often far from its optimum for health.

The crucial message is that not all carbs need to be avoided. But it is certainly advisable to steer clear of sugar and refined carbohydrates, and those with a high glycaemic index (GI) as explained below, as they are of little use to the body and can impose serious health risks.

WHAT IS THE GLYCAEMIC INDEX?

The glycaemic index (or GI) of a food is a system of ranking carbohydrate-containing foods and drinks according to how quickly they make blood sugar levels rise after eating them. Originally developed to help people with diabetes control their blood glucose levels, the GI is now widely used by everyone from dieters to sports people as a means of determining which foods will provide the longest lasting energy boost, thereby warding off hunger pangs and energy slumps. High-GI foods and drinks are quickly digested and cause a sharp rise in blood glucose levels

►

followed by a drop shortly afterwards. More preferable are low-GI foods, which are digested at a slower speed, making your blood glucose rise at a steady rate.

The GI of a food should be used as a general guide to healthy eating and not as a hard-and-fast rule for what is healthy and what is not. Foods with a high GI tend to be less favourable options, but are not necessarily unhealthy; for example, a baked potato has a high GI, whereas potato crisps – much higher in fat and salt – have a medium GI. Likewise, low-GI foods, perhaps surprisingly, include ice cream (which has its index lowered because it also contains protein) – not the best choice if you are trying to lose weight. All GI figures are a value given to the food when it is prepared on its own. Add milk, sugar or honey to porridge (a low-GI food) and it shifts the value somewhat.

The glycaemic load

Although the GI of a food is important, how much we eat of a food also has a huge influence of the effect it has on blood sugar. Eating a lot of a high GI food, such as white bread, will send blood sugar levels soaring. But it is difficult to eat large amounts of some high-GI foods, such as pineapple, which means the impact on blood sugar is unlikely to be as pronounced. It is on these principles that the concept of the glycaemic load (or GL) is based. The GL provides a value listed on the amount of a food you are likely to eat. Many foods that have high or medium GIs, such as kiwi fruit, pineapple and watermelon, can have low GLs. But the worst offenders in the high-GI stakes – white rice,

►

pasta, cornflakes and baked potato – are also likely to have high GLs. Tables of GL values are also available and many people consider them a more useful and practical measure of a food's effect on blood sugar than the GI tables.

To improve the GI of the food you eat, make the following swaps:

SWAP	FOR
White bread	Multigrain or wholemeal
Potatoes	Yam or sweet potato
White rice	Brown rice or basmati
Sugary breakfast cereals	Porridge
Overcooked soft pasta	Al dente pasta

Protein – the building block

If carbohydrates, or at least some of them, have been cast as nutritional baddies in recent years, then proteins have emerged from the dark side as unlikely heroes. Once chastised for being high in fat and causing muscle bulk – the antithesis of the dieter's dream – they are now considered key to successful weight loss.

Why protein is essential

It has always been known that proteins are essential for a healthy body. They are needed for muscle growth and repair and for maintenance of many of the body's structures. Proteins consist of molecules called amino acids; there are 22 amino acids needed for the body's functions, eight of which must be provided in the diet as they cannot be manufactured by the body. Protein that comes from animal sources – meat, fish, poultry, eggs and dairy products – provide all of the essential amino acids. Plant sources of protein – pulses, tofu, nuts, seeds and grains – lack some of the essential amino acids, so a good mix is needed if you eat a vegetarian diet or a diet low in meat and fish to ensure you get the variety needed.

Protein helps to control your appetite

Numerous studies have shown that protein-rich foods help you to feel full more quickly and this is part of the reason why many people now think the protein-to-carb ratio should shift in favour of protein foods when it comes to weight loss. When protein foods are consumed, messages are sent to the brain's satiation centres very quickly indicating that enough food has been eaten. Unlike sugary carbohydrates, proteins don't cause the kind of blood sugar spikes that lead to sugars in the bloodstream being retained as body fat.

The downside of too much protein

While proteins are gaining credence as the ultimate diet food, nutrition experts also know that extreme high-protein diets can be bad news. Cutting carbohydrates to very low levels triggers hypoglycaemia and the ketogenic state in which the body begins to rely on its own body fat for fuel, but this means that weakness and tiredness are the overwhelming result. When more protein is consumed than the body requires, the body responds by extracting the nitrogen part of a protein molecule and utilises the remaining carbon, oxygen and hydrogen as a source of calories. In the long term, high protein and very low-carb diets can cause digestive problems and are a risk for people with any kind of kidney disorder, so it's important to keep them in a healthy balance.

How to buy protein

Meals cooked from scratch are always the healthiest. Here's a quick guide to help you make the best protein choices.

Meat

For thousands of years, humans have relied on meats as an important part of the diet. Not only is it an important source of 'complete protein' (containing all eight of the essential amino acids the body needs to function) but it is also a key source of iron and other minerals. Studies have shown that meat-eating populations are at much less risk of iron-deficiency anaemia. Although red meat consumption has suffered from a succession of health scares in recent years, its image as a health threat is being challenged by emerging evidence that suggests that the fat it contains is not as harmful as previously thought (see page 25) and that the cholesterol contained in meat does not block arteries and actually plays a role in cell growth and the production of vitamin D.

Buying red meat can be a minefield, because much of the terminology used can be misleading; however, aiming for meat produced from grass-fed cattle is a good starting point according to research conducted at the University of Bristol.

Scientists there found that grass-fed beef retains its red colour for longer, a factor linked to the higher levels of the antioxidant vitamin E it contains. Grazed cattle also produced meat with significantly higher amounts of beneficial omega-3 fatty acids, some similar to those found in oily fish. From an ethical standpoint, too, grass-fed is best. Feeding cattle on grass throughout their lifecycle was shown to be the most environmentally sustainable way to rear beef, according to research for the National Trust.

Poultry

Chicken, turkey and other poultry provide a great source of protein in the diet and chicken is the UK's favourite meat source. Select poultry meats that are low in fat, such as turkey and chicken, and you have a meal that will leave you feeling satiated for much longer than a fatty carbohydrate snack. Although some forms of poultry – duck and goose, for example – are higher in fat, they also contain larger amounts of important minerals such as iron, vitamin B_{12} and selenium. When buying poultry, it is usually best to go for organic (although it comes with a hefty price premium) or at least check that the meat has not been 'bulked out' with added water or protein, a practice that is allowed but must be stated on food labelling.

Fish

Just one small portion – 100g (3½oz) – of fish provides between one-third and one-half of the protein an adult needs in a day. Fish is also a rich source of vitamin B_{12}, vital for a healthy nervous system, and iodine which the thyroid glands need to function effectively. Fatty fish, such as salmon and herrings, contain at least twice as many calories as white fish such as cod, but they also contain more of the omega oils that are beneficial to health (see page 29).

Modern fishing methods have resulted in a crisis in terms of fish availability and, consequently, many popular varieties of fish such as cod and plaice are now at least as expensive as meat. Less well-known types of white fish, such as coley, pollock and catfish, provide similar nutritional benefits at a lower cost. When buying seafood, such as prawns, beware that many frozen supplies have added salt or flavourings. Likewise, smoked fish is salted and seasoned, often with sugar, so always check labels before buying.

Vegetable protein

There are other sources of protein beyond those found in meat and dairy products. Many are usually described as 'incomplete proteins' because, unlike dairy foods and meat, they don't contain the eight essential amino acids required by the body for growth and maintenance; these are pulses (for example, lentils, kidney beans and chickpeas), nuts and seeds, although eggs, soya products, such as tofu and vegetable protein foods, are complete proteins. All are good sources of vegetarian protein. What's important if you are a non-meat eater is to ensure that you eat a variety of alternative protein foods so that you get all the essential amino acids (the 'building blocks') your body needs.

SOYA: WONDER-BEAN OR HAS-BEAN?

Soya is among the most popular forms of non-meat protein and, in recent years has been extolled as something of a wonder-bean if we eat enough of it. Research has shown that the plant hormones, or phytoestrogens, called isoflavones, it contains mimic the primary female sex hormone oestrogen and, as such, can lower cholesterol, reduce menopausal symptoms, boost bone density and even ward off the risks of some cancers; however, it is precisely these active compounds that have sparked growing dissent among some researchers.

What irks soya critics is that many of the positive and most widely publicised studies have been funded by the soya industry. And in the backlash against soya, less positive findings about the mass production of the bean are plentiful. Large quantities of the oestrogenic compounds have been shown to trigger premature puberty and increase the risk of other types of cancer. Researchers at the Queen Victoria Hospital in Belfast discovered soya consumption could have a profound adverse influence on male fertility. There are suggested links to thyroid problems and impaired endocrine function as well as reproductive development. In the UK, parents are advised not to feed infants soy formula before they are six months old.

Nevertheless, food manufacturers love the bean; it is cheap and incredibly versatile and, as such, has become ubiquitous in our food chain. It is estimated that 60 per cent of all processed foods sold in the UK contain soya in

►

some form. No fragment of the plant is discarded. Processed and refined, it can appear on ingredient labels as everything from soy protein isolate and textured vegetable protein to plant sterols. Oil extracted from soya is the most widely used in the world and, although often listed simply as 'vegetable oil' on packaging, is a common ingredient in margarines, spreads and salad dressings.

What of the Asian populations who eat large amounts of soya and appear to benefit from it? Purists who consume soya in the traditional forms – such as soy sauce, miso or tempeh – are not exposed to the side effects of harsh processing that are undertaken to produce mass quantities of soya. Traditional fermentation not only neutralises the naturally occurring toxins in the beans, making them more digestible, but it also reduces levels of isoflavones two to threefold. Industrial manufacturing methods do not have the same effect.

So how much soya, if any, is safe? Opinions vary as widely as the results of the studies into soya's effects. Most of the benefits have been shown with consistent intakes of a significant amount, around 25g (1oz), which would mean eating 2–3 portions of soya a day or 250ml (9fl oz) soya milk, a soya yoghurt and 100g (3½oz) of cooked soya beans or tofu. The safest recommendation seems to be to make sure soya is consumed in the unprocessed form such as miso or tempeh. Tofu and edamame beans are not fermented and should be eaten in small quantities. But the processed variety should be avoided. Soya is a mystery food we are beginning to understand.

Fat – the good and the bad

Fat finds itself in and out of fashion more frequently than flared trousers and leggings. One minute we are being urged to avoid it and are told that very low-fat diets are the way to go, the next minute fashionable diets, such as Atkins and Dukan, encourage us to gorge on it. Throughout its fluctuating popularity, there has been one constant: that saturated animal fats found in dairy foods are bad, bad, bad for the heart and we consume too much of them at our peril; however, even that accepted wisdom is now being touted as a big fat lie.

Not all fat is the same

There are three types of fat in the diet: saturated (mainly from animal sources), monounsaturated (such as olive oil) and polyunsaturated from plant sources and oily fish like mackerel and herrings. Nutritionists divide polyunsaturated fats, the healthiest type of fat, into two groups of what they call essential fatty acids (or EFAs): omega-3 and omega-6. It is crucial to include these fatty acids in the diet because they are found in every cell in the body but the body cannot produce them itself.

Until recently, it was saturated fat found in dairy foods and meat that got the bad rap. Its reputation appears to stem from studies that were carried out in the 1950s, 1960s and 1970s which showed that a high intake of animal fat not only raised cholesterol levels but was a strong predictor of heart attacks over a five-year period. The findings prompted medical experts around the world to change dietary recommendations to cut down on animal fats for the sake of your heart, and they are still heavily promoted today; however, the latest scientific research suggests that gaping holes existed in the research that lead to saturated fat being branded a killer.

In one of the landmark early studies, for example, researchers looked at animal fat consumption in seven countries. Although they found a high intake was a strong predictor of heart disease, the data wasn't rock solid, and in three of the countries studied there was no clear link. Other scientists have failed to show animal fat is as harmful as we are lead to believe. In one of the largest government-funded research programmes in the US, the Women's Health Initiative study, carried out at the Fred Hutchinson Cancer Research Center in Seattle in 2006, found that a diet low in total fat and saturated fat was shown to have no impact in reducing heart disease among the 20,000 women who took part.

A 77-page report by the British Nutrition Foundation challenged conventional wisdom about the effects of saturated fat in red meat. In the document, it was confirmed that there was 'no conclusive link' between cardiovascular disease and red meat. Repeated studies have shown that saturated fat has no adverse effect on blood cholesterol levels or other risk factors for cardiovascular disease. Indeed, it appears to be beneficial. One particular form of saturated fat, called stearic acid, which is found in beef and pork, skinless chicken, olive oil, cheese, chocolate and milk, now seems to deserve an especially clean bill of health because it may actually protect the heart against disease.

Stearic acid is one of many saturated fatty acids found in food and the main one present in red meat (others include lauric, myristic and palmitic acids). One study published in the *American Journal of Clinical Nutrition* revealed that eating lean beef on a daily basis improved the cholesterol levels of 42 subjects and found that it was the stearic acid in the meat that was responsible for the positive changes.

From butter to margarine and vegetable oils – a slippery path

What's more, over the last 30 years, the move away from satu-rated fat has had little or no effect on lowering the incidence of cardiovascular disease. What has happened instead is that people switched to margarines and spreads made from trans-fats, which have since been found to be more harmful than saturated fats ever were in promoting diabetes and heart problems. Added to that, the increased use of vegetable oil, soya and sunflower oils in place of saturated animal fats has lead to a higher consumption of the omega-6 oils they contain. Too much omega-6 oils (found in most edible oils, including sunflower and corn) can be detrimen-tal to health: a high intake prevents the body from metabolising omega-3 effectively, so cells can't carry electrical signals that are vital for optimal brain function effectively. Furthermore, one US study linked a high intake of omega-6 to the growth of prostate cancer cells in men. And in a UK survey of 14,500 families, preg-nant women with diets low in omega-3s and high in omega-6s were found to have an increased risk of depression.

Whereas people who eat omega-3-rich diets have neurones that run very fast, like Pentium-III microprocessors, those with too much omega-6 are slow and sluggish, like a 20-year-old silicon chip. Too much omega-6 has also been shown to increase the risk of arthritis by increasing inflammation of the joints and preventing the beneficial effects of omega-3 fatty acids from working.

The worst kind of fats: trans-fats

Of all fats used in modern food, trans-fats are public enemy number one. Scientists now know that trans-fats, created when liquid oils are put through a rigorous chemical hydrogenation process to transform them into solids, are more harmful to the heart and arteries than any fat from natural sources. Their use is widespread in the food industry and they are not only present in many margarines and spreads but in biscuits, cakes, crackers and ready meals as well as takeaways. They are cheap and tasty, but should be avoided. As well as being damaging to heart health, they appear to impinge on the brain's synapses, blocking communication signals and affecting concentration. As we will see later (page 89), manufacturers are not required to list trans-fats clearly on their labels, but look out for the words 'partially hydrogenated' or 'hydrogenated fats' on ingredient panels and put that food straight back on the shelf.

How much saturated fat is healthy?

The current recommended upper limit of saturated fat in the diet for women is a daily total of 20g (¾oz) and 30g (1oz) for men. Although these guidelines don't take into account the latest health evidence on fat science, the upper limit remains a useful guideline when it comes to weight maintenance. Myths and misconceptions have lead to consumers wrongly thinking that all saturated fat is bad when in fact they can eat sensible amounts of those rich in stearic acid, such as red meat, more than they probably realise.

So what conclusions can you make from this? Undoubtedly, the evidence against saturated fat found in dairy foods and meat is diminishing, and although not substantial enough to provide a green light for greater consumption of these important foods, it is sufficiently convincing for us to eat them without fear or panic and with the knowledge that they are better for us than many alternatives that are available, such as low-fat or convenience foods. Only when they are eaten in excess do they have the potential to cause harm, so stick within healthy limits.

Try not to eat too much omega-6s

It is the ratio of EFAs that we consume that is most important for health. The average diet has an omega-3 to omega-6 ratio of 1:10, whereas the recommended ratio is 1:3. So, although most people eat too much omega-6 – found in most vegetable oils, as described above – they are deficient in omega-3.

Eat more omega-3s

As we have seen, omega-3 fats provide significant health benefits. Scientists reporting in the *Journal of the American College of Cardiology* suggested that there is now 'compelling evidence' confirming the benefits of fish oils and suggested that everyone should consume more to obtain the omega-3 fatty acids they contain. Consuming two portions a week of oily fish, such as mackerel, herring and tuna, will help to supply a useful intake – a portion size is about 140g (5oz) of fish or one tuna steak, which would provide up to 250mg of omega-3 oils.

What are the gains? By far the strongest evidence in favour of fish oils is for heart health. Encouraging research, such as a study in the *Journal of the American College of Cardiology*, which documents convincing evidence that fish oils help to protect against repeated heart attacks in people with established heart disease, adds weight to the existing argument that omega-3 oils are helpful in preventing blood clotting and to regulate or lower blood pressure. It is thought that the fatty acids work inside the cell membranes, helping to boost the heart's electrical activity and to control blood pressure.

Much of the excitement about fish oil has centred on the use of supplements and their purported ability to enhance cognitive function. Consuming the fish oil fatty acid docosahexaenoic acid (DHA) has been shown to reduce the plaque formation in the brain that can lead to Alzheimer's disease and dementia, for example. There are several types of omega-3 fatty acids, but it is the long-chain omega-3 oils that provide the key substances DHA, thought to play a key role in the development of the infant brain, eye and vision development, and EPA (eicosapentaenoic acid) which also has a vital role in brain health.

Some researchers have also suggested that low omega-3 diets during pregnancy can result in children with more behaviour problems, such as ADHD; however, parents who routinely feed their children fish oil supplements may be surprised to learn that the evidence for omega-3 oils boosting intelligence and performance in exams is scant, whether they are supplied in supplement form or in fish. By far the strongest evidence in favour of omega-3 oils is that they boost heart health.

Most important is that we stick within the recommended limits for total fats (listed below) and cut out the trans-fats present in highly processed foods.

HOW MUCH FAT SHOULD WE EAT?

The current recommendation is to get no more than 35 per cent of your total calorie intake from fat and less than 10 per cent of that total should be saturated fat.

The recommended upper limit for adult women is a daily total of 70g (2½oz) of fat, 20g (¾oz) of which can be

▶

saturated; and for men 95g (3¼oz), 30g (1oz) of which can be saturated.

According to the traffic light system used in the UK (see below), a high-fat food contains more than 20g (¾oz) of fat per 100g (3½oz) of food; a low-fat food contains less than 5g (⅛oz) of fat per 100g (3½oz) of food.

TRAFFIC LIGHT SYSTEM

Red, amber and green traffic light colours are used voluntarily by some food manufacturers on packaging in the UK. They tell you about the levels of fat, salt and sugar in food.

- **Red** signals that the food is high in fat, salt or sugar.

- **Amber** means that the food has medium quantities of fat, salt or sugar, and is a reasonable choice for a meal.

- **Green** signals that the food contains low amounts of fat, salt or sugar, and is healthy to eat.

Most foods will have a mixture of traffic light colours, and the advice is to go for those that are predominantly green. Traffic lights are a useful guide, but it is also important to check the backs of packs and the ingredient panels for more detailed information.

Olive oil

When it comes to vegetable oils, the best choice is olive oil, in particular extra virgin, the purest form. Comprising mainly of monounsaturated omega-9 fatty acids, which are heart-protective, it has been linked to lower levels of heart disease and protection against high blood pressure and cholesterol levels. It is also rich in vitamin E, other antioxidants and plant compounds that are linked to disease protection, and it is one of the reasons the Mediterranean diet is so healthy. Olive oil is not heat stable at high temperatures, however, so it is not suitable for frying. It can be bought in a spray, which makes it handy for adding a fine layer when low-fat cooking or using a toaster.

Fibre – adding bulk

Most of us know that fibre plays an important role in the diet, but because the terms used to describe it are confusing, its benefits are often misunderstood. Of the two main types, soluble fibre dissolves in water; insoluble fibre does not. This key difference determines how each type of fibre acts in the body to benefit your health. Most foods contain both forms. But most people in the West don't consume enough fibre to benefit health. According to the UK's National Health Service, average fibre consumption is about 14g (½oz) of fibre a day – the target is at least 18g (¾oz) daily.

A growing trend in the food industry is to add fibre to foods that don't necessarily contain any naturally. This so-called 'functional fibre' is isolated and extracted from plants or animal sources and added to drinks and foods to boost their fibre content. Although it is better than nothing, getting fibre from whole foods is infinitely preferable, as they contain many other healthful plant compounds. Here's a quick run-down of where to get fibre and the boost it can give:

Soluble fibre Found in oatmeal and oat bran, oats, lentils, apples, oranges, pears, strawberries, blueberries, nuts, flaxseed, beans and peas, cucumbers, celery and carrots, this type of fibre draws in water and forms a gel, which slows down digestion. By delaying the emptying of your stomach, it makes you feel full, which, in turn, helps to control your weight. It is known that slower stomach emptying also affects blood sugar levels and has a positive effect on insulin sensitivity and the prevention of type-2 diabetes. It is also the type of fibre that has a prebiotic effect, which means it helps to create and maintain levels of gut-friendly bacteria (see page 98).

Insoluble fibre Found in whole wheat, whole grains, seeds, nuts, barley, brown rice, bulgur, celery, broccoli, cabbage, onions, tomatoes, carrots, cucumbers, green beans, root vegetable skins, dark leafy vegetables, raisins, grapes and other fruits. Because it does not dissolve in water, it passes through the gastrointestinal tract relatively intact to speed up the passage of food and waste through your gut. It has a laxative effect and adds bulk to the diet, helping prevent constipation.

Salt – why we need only a small amount

Sodium chloride, or salt, is an element essential for health. Every cell in the body needs it to function – it is required to regulate fluid balance and for nerves and muscles, such as those in the heart, to function well. Too little salt can cause mental confusion, an inability to concentrate and, in extreme cases, the potentially fatal condition hyponatraemia which leads to body salts becoming dangerously diluted followed by the brain swelling beyond the skull's capacity.

Not that salt depletion is a risk for most of us. Although

intake has fallen as food manufacturers have begun to add less salt to food, the latest figures show that the average person still consumes 8.6g of salt a day – that's 0.9g less than in 2000–2001, but not low enough. From the day you are born, your blood pressure starts to rise slowly. Salt is a major factor in that increase, and high-salt diets are thought to be the main reason why blood pressure rises with age. Precisely how salt raises blood pressure is not entirely clear, but it is thought that when salt intake is too high, the kidneys struggle to pass it all into the urine and some ends up in the bloodstream. This then draws more water into the blood, increasing volume and pressure.

The long-term goal of health campaigners is to have adults cut salt to 6g daily, a total of around one teaspoon, and children need even less. Most people could do with cutting down. A study in the *Journal of Human Hypertension*, which looked at the salt intakes of 1,658 children in the UK aged 7–18 found salt to be responsible for raising blood pressure in children. The problem is that it's not that easy to remove salt from the diet. Adding it at the dinner table accounts for only a tiny fraction (about 5 per cent) of the total salt we consume on a daily basis. Much of it is hidden in the highly processed food many people now eat in such large amounts; indeed, breakfast cereals and desserts can contain more salt than a bag of crisps. Some takeaway meals contain double the amount of salt an adult is recommended to consume in a day.

How to control your salt intake

Finding out how much salt is in your food can be confusing, because manufacturers may list a food's *sodium* content or its *salt* content, or sometimes both. In the food swaps that follow, the *salt* content of a food will be listed, but when you are food swapping yourself, there is a simple calculation that you can use to convert sodium levels into salt levels:

sodium grams multiplied by 2.5 = salt grams

Choose foods that enable you to stick within the healthy guidelines below.

Daily salt recommendations:

0–6 months: 1g

7–12 months: 1g

1–3 years: 2g

4–6 years: 3g

7–10 years: 5g

11–14 years: 6g

Adults: 6g

Guidelines in the UK state that a high-salt food contains over 1.5g of salt per 100g (3½oz). A low-salt food contains no more than 0.3g of salt per 100g (3½oz).

Sugar – not quite so sweet

For years we knew that too much of the sweet stuff would make us put on weight and rot our teeth, but, of the terrible trio – sugar, fat and salt – it seemed to be the one in which we could indulge with slightly less of a guilty conscience. After all, it is a natural source of energy, the kind of carbohydrate that was used by athletes to fuel their bodies. We could do worse than satisfy our sweet tooth once in a while – or could we?

Experts are now so concerned about our increasing fondness for sugary foods that they are issuing stark warnings about the effects of sugar overload on our health. A report published in *Circulation*, the journal of the American Heart Association (AHA), linked a high intake of the sweet stuff not only to obesity but everything from raised blood pressure to heart disease and strokes. It is known to cause dental problems and has even been linked to cancer as well as a number of other illnesses. One European study found that women with the highest blood sugar levels increased their risk of cancers of the pancreas, skin, womb and urinary tract by as much as 26 per cent.

When sugar and sugary foods are eaten, the response is a sharp rise in levels of glucose (sugar) in the bloodstream which forces the pancreas to pump out insulin, the hormone needed to keep blood sugar levels under control. Insulin's job is to extract glucose from the bloodstream, convert it into glycogen and store it in the liver or muscles; however, since the body has only a limited storage capacity for glycogen, excess glucose from sugars and refined carbs is then stashed away as fat, eventually causing related health issues.

How much is the most we should eat?

Guideline daily amounts set by the UK government suggest women restrict their total sugar intake, including natural sugars, which are locked within the cells of fruit and vegetables, to 90g (3¼oz) and men to 120g (4¼oz). When it comes to so-called 'extrinsic sugars', those that are added to food during manufacture or preparation, the advice is for men to eat no more than 65g (2¼oz) and women no more than 50g (1¾oz) a day. According to the UK guidelines on sugar, a high-sugar food contains over 15g (½oz) of sugar per 100g (3½oz); a low-sugar food contains 5g (⅛oz) of sugar or less per 100g (3½oz) of food. For this reason it is best to limit fruit to no more than three of your 'five-a-day'.

In the US, men are advised to take no more than 150 calories (9 teaspoons) worth of sugars added to food and drink and women no more than 100 (6 teaspoons) every day. But those levels are considered upper limits and in reality it is best to opt for foods that have no added sugar and not to over-consume even naturally sugary foods such as dried fruit. Around the world we are all being urged to consume less of the sweet stuff, yet, most of us are failing dismally to stick to these levels. Since the 1980s, sugar consumption in the UK has increased by almost one-third to 550g (1¼lb) per person per week, an amount that exceeds the healthy guidelines by a huge margin. People now get almost one-fifth of their calories from sugar.

The hidden dangers

With fewer of us adding sugar to our tea and coffee, how are we amassing these individual sugar mountains? The answer is: hidden sugars in the food we buy. It is easy to see how upper limits are reached when you consider that a single can of cola contains 7 teaspoons of sugar and an organic, tomato-based pasta sauce has 2 teaspoons per serving. And it is no longer just sucrose, or table sugar, that we need to look out for. Sugars come from cane, beet or corn. Virtually anything ending in the letters 'ose' is likely to be a sugar. Of particular concern are new forms of high-calorie sweeteners that are cheaply made and widely used, such as high-fructose corn syrup or HFCS (see page 196). Honey and syrups are also sweeteners and count towards our daily levels.

How food is labelled

Understanding food labels is key to successful food swapping, but they can be a mystery to fathom and they often don't tell you exactly the information you might expect. Reading food labels is almost like learning a foreign language: with practice you soon become adept at translating what seems incomprehensible at first. The key is to look at values per 100g (3½oz) as opposed to serving sizes. With this information you can then cross-refer between different brands to find out which provides the best nutrient profile.

By looking at the values per 100g (3½oz) you will have an indication of the percentage of sugar, fat and salt that a product contains; for example, a packet of biscuits containing 21.2g of sugar per 100g (3½oz) means that 21.2 per cent of its weight is sugar.

Guideline Daily Amounts (GDAs)

To help you further, here is a guide to labelling terms that are most commonly used in the UK. Some manufacturers use these in place of the voluntary traffic light system (see page 31). GDAs are a guide to how many calories and nutrients we can safely consume in a day; however, they are intended to be a guideline rather than a target that we should aim to meet. Children have different GDAs to adults (as listed in the charts opposite) until they reach age 18. In most cases, we should aim to consume less (and definitely not more) than the GDAs for fat, salt and sugar.

The GDAs for adults

Food group	Women	Men
Calories	2,000	2,500
Protein	45g	55g
Carbohydrate	230g	300g
Sugars	90g	120g
Fat	70g	95g
Saturated fat	20g	30g
Fibre	24g	24g
Salt	6g	6g

The GDAs for children from 5 to 18 years

Food group	Children 5–10 years	Girls 11–14 years	Boys 11–14 years
Calories	1,800	1,850	2,200
Protein	24g	41g	42g
Carbohydrate	220g	230g	275g
Sugar	85g	90g	110g
Fat	70g	70g	85g
Saturated fat	20g	25g	25g
Fibre	14g	15g	15g
Salt	4g	6g	6g

Food group	Girls 15–18 years	Boys 15–18 years
Calories	2,100	2,750
Protein	45g	55g
Carbohydrate	265g	345g
Sugar	105g	140g
Fat	80g	105g
Saturated fat	25g	35g
Fibre	24g	24g
Salt	6g	6g

CHECK THE LABEL

When buying breakfast cereals, check the label for the sugar content in the table marked 'typical values per 100g'. Although most manufacturers also provide a 'per serving' figure, the amounts are based on a portion size that is far smaller than the average bowlful and so does not give an accurate representation. Check the figure listed under 'Carbohydrates, of which sugars' in the 'per 100g' values: if it is higher than 15g (or 15 per cent), then you are holding a high sugar product. Best put it back on the shelf.

What the descriptive words on packaging mean

Some words in packaging can be helpful whereas others can't be relied upon to tell you anything useful about the food you are buying. It's worth understanding what manufacturers mean when they use certain terms. The following terms are used in the UK:

Pure, fresh, authentic, original, farmhouse, home-made and traditional are all words that you can ignore. Manufacturers tend to be economical with the truth when describing their products, and the terms have no legal meaning.

Sell-by/best-before dates Sell-by dates are for shop staff rather than shoppers, and best-before dates relate to quality and not safety. Foods consumed past these dates are likely to be safe to eat. Eggs, for example, can be eaten a few days after their best-before date.

Use-by date This term is used on perishable foods and those sold in the chiller cabinets. It's advisable to stick to these dates and not consume the food after the use-by date on a label.

Light/lite A food must be 30 per cent lower in a particular value (calories, fat or sugar) than a standard version of the product to be classified as light or lite. It doesn't mean much, unfortunately, because a light chocolate mousse can still be high in sugar and calories – it might just be lower in fat.

Low fat A product must contain no more than 3g of fat per 100g (3½oz) of food or 1.5g of fat per 100ml (3½fl oz) of liquid.

No added sugar/unsweetened doesn't mean that a food is sugar-free. In the case of 'no added sugar', a food can still contain sugar, but it must not have been added as an ingredient. Likewise, 'unsweetened' means that no sugars or sweeteners have been added, but those naturally present can still make the food very sweet.

With a basic understanding of the language used in the labelling of foods and the kinds of levels of nutrients we are seeking for healthy eating, you can now use the swaps and choices in the following chapters to help you to shop wisely whether for weight loss or to maintain a healthy weight.

CHAPTER **THREE**

.

Store-cupboard Foods

YOU MIGHT THINK THE BASIC supplies you buy on a weekly basis have always been the same, but it's not always the case. Foodstuffs that have been around for centuries – eggs and bread, for example – have changed beyond recognition in the way that they are produced or manufactured. Ingredients we had never heard of 20 or 30 years ago are thrown into the mix, sometimes to the benefit of you, the consumer, but often not. This chapter looks at some of the most commonly used and popular of the store-cupboard basics with tips on how to swap for maximum effect.

Bread

After decades of plummeting sales in which bread consumption dropped by 35 per cent because of concerns that it caused weight gain and bloating, sales of loaves are on the up for the first time in almost 30 years. Evidence of our renewed love affair with the loaf can be seen everywhere, with artisan bakeries selling loaves as far removed from a polythene-packed white sliced as you could imagine cropping up on high streets and in shopping centres faster than you could toast a couple of slices. But the swell in sales is only one side of bread's success story. Scientists are also backing its re-emergence as a fashionable food with solid evidence that it should never have been billed the unpopular food item it became.

Gram for gram, bread has fewer than half the calories of fat, it's packed with B vitamins and if you choose wholemeal or fruit breads you get plenty of fibre, which is important for digestion and bowel health. Four slices of wholemeal bread provides almost half your daily fibre requirement. Add walnuts, dried fruit, seeds and grains, and the range of vitamins and minerals soars.

The anti-bread crusade was exacerbated by several studies that appeared to link the food to a raised risk of disease. Eating more than 2 slices of white bread a day was associated with an increased likelihood of diabetes in a study by the Cancer Council of Australia, and the highly refined carbohydrates in white bread have also been linked to a raised risk of heart disease in women. However, the relationship is weak and it has never been proven that bread itself is directly responsible for ill-health, only too many refined carbohydrates.

Much of bread's other bad press in the past stemmed from the manufacturing methods in its mass production. Most 'sliced and wrapped', or 'fake, plastic' bread, which still accounts for about 76 per cent of that sold, is churned out on a massive industrial scale and uses a number of chemical 'improvers' designed to shorten production time, plus preservatives to prolong shelf life. An ingredients panel on loaf packaging with a lengthy list of enzyme-softening agents and emulsifiers, along with scare stories about the high levels of salt in pre-packaged bread (4 slices of some varieties provide almost half the recommended daily intake of sodium) have wrestled with our healthy-eating conscience.

Getting the best out of your bread

All bread is not equal. Speciality breads can contain hidden calories and fat. Delicious though they are, be careful what you choose.

SWAP ▸ Soft white medium sliced

Per slice: calories 96; fat 0.9g; sugars 1.4g; salt 0.42g

This is a typical white sliced loaf with not much going for it on the nutritional front. It has medium amounts of salt.

FOR ▸ Wholemeal sliced

Per slice: calories 93; fat 1.0g; sugars 1.5g; salt 0.44g

The advantage here is not calories, fat or salt content but the fact that wholemeal contains more fibre than white which is important for a healthy bowel and digestive system. If you must have sliced, this is the type to choose. Be aware that 'stay fresh' versions of sliced bread contain more preservatives.

––––––––––

SWAP ▸ Tiger top

Per slice: calories 142; fat 2.5g; sugars 1.6g; salt 0.4g

A tiger top *pain de mie* loaf, characterised by its mottled crust, has butter and eggs added, which bump up the fat content. The cracked crust is, in fact, the result of a glaze made from olive oil and sugar.

FOR ▶ Sourdough

Per slice: calories 120; fat 0.3g; sugars 1.3g; salt 0.3g

Made without yeast, it uses what is known as a 'starter': a mixture of flour and water that is soured through a fermentation process. The gas produced by fermentation is trapped inside the elastic gluten structure of the dough and causes it to rise. The process produces natural probiotic substances that are thought to be beneficial for the digestion. You save 20 calories per slice compared to the tiger top loaf.

––––––––

SWAP ▶ Ciabatta

Per slice: calories 120; fat 2.1g; sugars 1.0g; salt 0.4g

Ciabatta is generally made with at least 4 per cent olive oil, which increases the fat and calorie content. Soak it in olive oil and you are looking at almost 200 calories per slice.

FOR ▶ Irish soda

Per slice: calories 82; fat 1.3g; sugars 2.3g; salt 0.4g

A yeast-free variety of bread that is useful for those with an intolerance to yeast. Soda bread uses bicarbonate of soda as a raising agent. The bicarbonate of soda reacts with another ingredient, buttermilk, and makes the bread rise. It is a good choice, especially if made with wholemeal flour, and saves almost 60 calories.

––––––––

SWAP ▸ Garlic flatbread

Per slice: calories 155; fat 4.7g; sugars 1.6g; salt 0.5g

Because it contains a substantial amount of olive oil, this flat-bread falls into the medium category for fat, so it's not the best choice. Even worse would be the cheese-topped garlic flatbread that is available.

FOR ▸ Pepper focaccia

Per slice: calories 130; fat 3.1g; sugars 2.0g; salt 0.6g

This olive oil-infused bread contains peppers, which add a little vitamin C and fibre. It is among the highest in terms of its salt content per slice, but has fewer calories and fat than the flatbread.

———

SWAP ▸ Multigrain sliced batch

Per slice: calories 140; fat 4.3g; sugars 1.9g; salt 0.5g

This is very different from the kind of multigrain you might get from a bakery, which would contain a combination of flours that contain close to the complete grain, including wheat germ, kibbled grains, whole grains and usually seeds such as sunflower and sesame. The sliced version is often just wholegrain, barley malt and wheat bran with sugar added for sweetness.

FOR ▸ Rye

Per slice: calories 90; fat 0.6g; sugars 1.2g; salt 0.4g

Made with flour produced from the rye kernel, rye bread has a dark colour from the caramelisation of the starch in the grain and a dense texture, which makes it filling. A study in the *Journal of Nutrition* showed rye bread to be more effective at maintaining bowel regularity than wheat bread. It's also low GI, releasing sugars more slowly into the bloodstream for sustained energy. Plus it saves you 50 calories per slice.

WATCH OUT FOR SALT

The salt content of bread has caused concern for many years, and while some manufacturers have made steps towards reducing it, surveys show that one in four shop-bought loaves contain as much salt in a single slice as a packet of crisps. Among the worst culprits are expensive artisan breads sold in bakeries, which often have no packaging and labelling. When the lobby group Consensus Action on Salt and Health conducted their most recent research into the salt levels of popular breads, they discovered that one particular artisan bread had 2.83g of salt per 100g (3½oz), almost half the total recommended daily intake. Of packaged breads, a healthy-sounding seeded farmhouse loaf had the most with 2.03g per 100g (3½oz).

Crackers and crispbreads

Once, crackers and crispbreads were dull, cardboard-tasting snacks that did little to tempt the palate unless a slab of cheese was plonked on top. In much the same way as the bread market, though, the crackers scene has exploded so that we are now offered a huge range of highly tempting variations on the original theme.

Of course, the type and amount of cheese you consume with your cracker will have a big influence on the overall calorie and fat content of your snack, but selecting your crackers wisely is also important. Many contain hidden fat and, like bread, relatively high amounts of salt.

Bear in mind that cracker sizes vary enormously and some are half the size of others, which means you'd probably end up eating more of them before you are full.

SWAP ▶ Jacob's Hovis digestive

Per biscuit: calories 37; fat 2.2g; sugars 2.2g; salt trace

Digestives look wholesome but are often highly sweetened and over-refined so that they contain little fibre. In this case, the biscuits contain both sugar and glucose syrup – unnecessary in a savoury biscuit intended for cheese.

FOR ▶ Jacob's cream crackers

Per cracker: calories 35; fat 1.1g; sugars 0.1g; salt 0.1g

Cream crackers remain the best selling of all crackers and crisp-breads. Made with wheat flour, vegetable oil, salt and yeast, they are low in fibre but also relatively low in calories and contain half the fat of the digestive.

––––––––––

SWAP ▶ Ryvita golden rye crackers for cheese

Per crispbread: calories 27; fat 0.2g; sugars 2.2g; salt trace

A variation on the original Ryvita theme. It is easy to eat several of these small circular crackers (they weigh just 7g each), which would mean that you could quickly exceed 100 calories before adding butter or cheese.

FOR ▶ Carr's melts originals

Per cracker: calories 20; fat 0.9g; sugars 0.3g; salt trace

Not the healthiest in terms of fibre and nutritional profile, but these biscuits offer a saving of 7 calories per biscuit over the Ryvita version. They also contain much less sugar.

———————

SWAP ▶ Tuc cheese sandwich

Per cracker: calories 72; fat 4.3g; sugars 0.5g; salt 0.2g

This is a highly refined and over-processed biscuit sandwiched together with a mixture made from dried, powdered cheese. The biscuits are sweetened with glucose syrup and contain whey powder for added bulk. With 31 per cent fat they have a high fat content and are in the medium category for salt – 1.5g per 100g (3½oz).

FOR ▶ McVitie's cheddars

Per cracker: calories 20; fat 1.2g; sugars 0.2g; salt 0.1g

These contain similar ingredients to the Tuc sandwich and they are also sweetened, in this case with both sugar and glucose syrup. But they lack the filing, which lowers the calorie and fat content considerably. If it's a cheese flavour you are after, these will save you 52 calories a biscuit.

———————

SWAP ▶ Ritz original crackers

Per 4 biscuits: calories 62; fat 3.2g; sugars 0.8g; salt 0.4g

These biscuits are tiny, and the manufacturer suggests a serving size is 8 crackers – double the amount listed here, which means 123 calories. A serving of 8 provides 13 per cent of your daily salt intake. Sweetened with glucose syrup and sugar, there is not much in them that is particularly nutritionally beneficial.

FOR ▶ Nairn's rough oatcakes

Per biscuit: calories 45; fat 2.0g; sugars 0.1g; salt 0.1g

Containing only oats, oil and salt, these are among the few biscuits not to contain added sugar in some form. Oats are high in soluble fibre, which produces a slow and sustained release of carbohydrates in the form of energy. In short, 1 or 2 of these are a healthier choice than crackers made with refined white flour. And they compare extremely favourably to the Ritz.

––––––––––

SWAP ▶ Dr Karg organic Emmenthal and pumpkin seed crispbreads

Per crispbread: calories 107; fat 3.7g; sugars 0.2g; salt 0.5g

Granted, these crispbreads are big (25g per slice) and are loaded with 16 per cent organic seeds including pumpkin, sunflower, linseed and sesame, which are filling and contain healthy fats as well as protein. You'd be better off eating the seeds as a snack on their own than on top of a crispbread. The oil in the seeds bumps up the fat content meaning you could quickly tot up several hundred calories once cheese is added.

FOR ▶ Ryvita pumpkin seeds and oat crispbread

Per crispbread: calories 44; fat 0.9g; sugars 0.6g; salt 0.07g

With less than half the calories and about one-quarter of the fat content per slice, these rye crispbreads provide you with 20 per cent pumpkin seeds to fill you up as well as 16 per cent oats. They are much lower in salt than many other crackers.

————————

SWAP ▸ Jacob's salt and cracked black pepper flatbread

Per portion: calories 41; fat 0.8g; sugars 0.3g; salt 0.1g

These flatbreads contain vegetable oil, poppy seeds and flavourings. They may be tasty, but you can slash the calories in half if you choose a healthier option.

FOR ▸ Finn Crisp original slims

Per cracker: calories 20; fat 0.1g; sugars 0.1g; salt 0.2g

Made from 94 per cent wholegrain rye with no oil added, these are the ultimate low-calorie crispbread and a good source of fibre to boot (1.2g per slice); however, like the Jacob's version, they are small and it would be easy to eat several in one sitting.

Dried fruit and nuts

Nibbling on nuts and dried fruits has a healthy image, but it should be done with caution if you are trying to lose weight. Nuts are composed of heart-friendly omega oils and are among the richest sources of omega-9 oils as well as being an important provider of bone-building calcium and protein, which helps to regenerate muscle and tissue fibres, but they do come with a fairly hefty calorie price to pay. The good news is that scientists have found that eating nuts seems to leave people feeling fuller more quickly so that they are less likely to snack on other foods, but too high an intake will undoubtedly lead to piling on extra pounds.

Similarly, dried fruits are a great snack – in moderation. They are generally high in fibre, iron and potassium. Unfortunately they are also high in sugar. Dried fruit doesn't magically acquire extra calories, it just loses up to 90 per cent of its water content and this concentrates the sugar that is naturally present in the fruit. So whereas one dried apricot has exactly the same calorie count and much the same nutritional content as a fresh one, it just weighs a lot less and is smaller, so it's easy to eat a lot more.

Both dried fruits and nuts are best bought in their unadulterated state. Adding salt, flavourings, chocolate or other coatings will offset the benefits provided by the original foodstuff to a large extent. Enjoy them – sparingly.

SWAP ▶ Ocean Spray craisins

Per 100g (3½oz) serving: calories 319; fat 1.4g; sugar 65.0g; salt trace

These are the latest take on traditional raisins – dried cranberries, sweetened with sugar and with oil added during the manufacturing process.

FOR ▶ Raisins

Per 100g (3½oz) serving: calories 289; fat 0.5g; sugar 69.0g; salt trace

Raisins are the most convenient low-fat snack. They are made from dried grapes and are a good source of iron and potassium (a handful provides 7 per cent of the recommended intake). Although they aren't a low-calorie snack, they are low in fat and, unlike craisins, they are naturally sweet and don't contain added sugar. Save yourself 30 calories with the swap.

———

SWAP ▶ Luxury fruit and nuts mix

Per 100g (3½oz) serving: calories 456; fat 35.4g; sugar 24.5g; salt trace

This mix comprises raisins, almonds, pistachio nuts, Brazil nuts, cashew nuts, pecan nuts and cranberries. A 30g (1oz) handful supplies a fifth of the recommended daily amount of vitamin E. Beware of the addition of chocolate chips to a mix like this. The fat comes from the oil in the nuts and it's easy to consume several hundred calories as you nibble on the delicious mix. Best reserved for an occasional treat.

FOR ▶ Organic dried apricots

Per 100g (3½oz) serving: calories 285; fat 0.5g; sugar 34.5g; salt trace

Non-organic dried apricots are often treated with the chemical sulphur dioxide to preserve their bright orange colour; however, its addition is unnecessary and the chemical can trigger allergic reactions, including asthma, in some people or cause gastrointestinal discomfort in others. Those that don't contain sulphur dioxide tend to be a darker colour. They are an excellent source of potassium and a good source of iron. Plus they contain 144 fewer calories per 100g (3½oz) than the luxury mix.

––––––

SWAP ▶ Banana chips

Per 100g (3½oz) serving: calories 525; fat 31.0g; sugar 22.2g; salt trace

Don't be fooled into thinking that banana chips are a healthy fruit alternative. Just over half the weight is actually the fruit itself. The rest comes from coconut oil and sugar. Although pure and unrefined coconut oil is no longer considered a health villain in liquid form as it was in the 1980s – the main saturated fat it contains, lauric acid, is a medium-chain fatty acid that doesn't affect cholesterol levels adversely in the way once thought – the coconut oil used commercially is often chemically treated and partially hydrogenated creating the dreaded trans-fats that are known to have health risks. A handful has more saturated fat than two cupcakes, outweighing any goodness. Even worse is the 'yoghurt-coated' variety, which is very high in fat and sugar. You'd be better off with a bag of sweets.

FOR ▶ Medjool dates

Per 100g (3½oz) serving: calories 295; fat 0.1g; sugar 62.8g; salt trace

Both fresh and dried dates make a great snack – expect about double the calories on a weight-for-weight basis in the dried version such as these. Medjool dates are the so-called kings of the date world because of their size and sweetness. They have a toffee-like texture, and are rich in potassium, fibre, magnesium and copper. They do contain about 60 calories each, so be careful how many you consume. Still, you save 230 calories per 100g (3½oz) compared to sugar-laden banana chips.

––––––––––

SWAP ▶ Brazil nuts

Per 100g (3½oz) serving: calories 682; fat 68g; sugar 2.4g; salt trace

Brazil nuts are rich in selenium, which helps to protect and build the body's cells. Just 3–4 of the nuts a day will meet a woman's needs for this mineral. Raised selenium intakes have been linked to a reduced risk of certain cancers, such as lung and prostate; however, Brazil nuts are among the most calorific, so treat yourself only occasionally.

FOR ▸ Almonds

Per 100g (3½oz) serving: calories 629; fat 55.8g; sugar 4.2g; salt trace

A slight saving on calories here, but there may be other advantages for the swap. Researchers have shown that women who consumed 40 almonds a day didn't gain weight after a six-month trial. It could be that not all the fat in almonds is absorbed by the body. They are high in magnesium and calcium. A worthy exchange.

———————

SWAP ▸ Walnuts

Per 100g (3½oz) serving: calories 696; fat 68.5g; sugar 2.6g; salt trace

Walnuts are a nutrient-dense food, with high levels of the minerals manganese and copper, as well as an antioxidant compound called ellagic acid that helps to block the metabolic processes causing inflammation, which can lead to insulin resistance and diabetes. Eating about 30g (1oz) of the nuts a day was shown to lower cholesterol levels by an average of 0.3 points in one study. A good choice for health benefits; however, there are lower-calorie options.

FOR ▸ Cashew nuts

Per 100g (3½oz) serving: calories 588; fat 43.9g; sugar 5.9g; salt trace

Often overlooked in the health stakes, plain cashew nuts (avoid the salted and flavoured varieties) are packed with iron, containing double the amount of many other nuts and with twice the concentration present in minced beef. Just 25 cashew nuts a day provides the level of iron required by an adult woman. They also contain 108 fewer calories than walnuts, so they make a perfect snack.

Condiments and salad dressings

To many people, eating a salad with no dressing, chips without ketchup or a sandwich without mayonnaise is unthinkable. Yet it's worth calculating how many extra calories and added fat are loaded into a meal or snack when you pour or spoon on a sauce. The good news is that many are highly flavoured, and this means that you don't need much to make a difference in terms of taste – but those extra spoonfuls soon add up.

SWAP ▶ Heinz tomato ketchup

Per 100g (3½oz): calories 103; fat 0.1g; sugars 23.7g; salt 2.2g

Traditional tomato ketchup is high in both sugar and salt. It contains about 20 calories per tablespoon, about the amount you would put on a hot dog. On the plus side, it is a good source of lycopene, an antioxidant substance in tomatoes that is absorbed by the body more effectively when it is processed or cooked, as it is here. High intakes of lycopene have been shown to prevent cancer and slow the disease as well as lowering the risk of heart disease.

FOR ▶ Heinz reduced-sugar tomato ketchup

Per 100g (3½oz): calories 77; fat 0.1g; sugars 16.3g; salt 1.7g

Having cottoned on to the fact that consumers are balking at the large amounts of sugar added to ketchup, many manufacturers have cut down the quantities and made versions such as this. It does offer considerably less sugar (16 per cent) and cuts calories to 13 per spoon, but it is still not a low-sugar food.

————————

SWAP ▸ Hellmann's real mayonnaise

Per 100g (3½oz): calories 722; fat 79.1g; sugars 1.3g; salt 1.5g

Among the most popular ingredients in sandwiches, mayonnaise – made with oil and eggs – is notoriously calorie-laden. A tablespoon typically contains 138 calories and 15g of fat – almost 80 per cent of the content of this mayonnaise is fat.

FOR ▸ Hellmann's extra–light mayonnaise

Per 100g (3½oz): calories 73; fat 3g; sugars 4.8g; salt 2.75g

With only 3 per cent fat, this offers a considerable saving on the full-fat version. It also contains 70 per cent fewer calories, but avoid slapping it on too heartily – its salt content is high.

————————

SWAP ▸ Pizza Express Caesar light

Per 100ml (3½fl oz): calories 348; fat 34.1g; sugars 6.8g; salt 2.2g

For a product that is labelled 'light', this is tremendously high in fat and calories. The high calories come mainly from the 30 per cent rapeseed oil it contains. It's also high in salt.

FOR ▸ Tesco finest Caesar

Per 100g (3½oz): calories 300; fat 28.1g; sugars 2.9g; salt 1.0g

Not a particularly low-fat option, but this Caesar dressing offers a saving in fat, calories and salt compared to the 'light'

Pizza Express version. All creamy-based dressings – ranch, blue cheese and Caesar – are higher in fat than many others, so use sparingly.

SWAP ▶ Newman's Own balsamic dressing

Per 100g (3½oz): calories 326; fat 33.3g; sugars 3.0g; salt 1.7g

The main ingredient here is rapeseed oil (although it also contains 3 per cent olive oil), which accounts for the fact that one-third of the weight is fat and earns it a high-fat status. There is 17 per cent balsamic vinegar but it also contains sugar.

FOR ▶ Balsamic vinegar

Per 100ml (3½fl oz): calories 90; fat 0g; sugars 16.9g; salt trace

Balsamic vinegar is made with wine vinegar and grape must concentrate and contains no fat. It makes a great salad dressing because you need to use very little of it – a large spoonful contains only 20 calories. The perfect switch.

SWAP ▶ HP brown sauce

Per 100g (3½oz): calories 129; fat 0.1g; sugars 23.5g; salt 2.1g

Tomatoes and malt vinegar are the main ingredients in this brown sauce with dates, spices and flavourings giving it the tangy edge; however, it is also sweetened with fructose syrup and sugar, which means it is classified as a high-sugar food.

FOR ▶ Daddies brown sauce

Per 100g (3½oz): calories 108; fat trace; sugars 18.4g;
salt 2.0g

This has the edge on calories and sugar alone. It contains no
tomatoes and is also sweetened with HFCS and sugar so not
the perfect line up of ingredients. But you do save a few calories
per spoonful.

––––––––––

SWAP ▶ Branston tomato and red pepper relish

Per 100g (3½oz): calories 160; fat 0.4g; sugars 34.9g;
salt 1.2g

Relishes are generally the accompaniment of choice for burgers.
The most prevalent ingredient in this product is sugar, which
explains why well over one-third of its weight comes from the
sweet stuff. It also contains artificial sweeteners.

FOR ▶ Levi Roots mango and chilli relish

Per 100g (3½oz): calories 110; fat 0.2g; sugars 20.2g;
salt 0.75g

This is sweetened with sugar (as are most relishes and chutneys)
as well as pineapples in syrup and pineapple juice concentrate,
but the main ingredient is water followed by low-calorie malt
vinegar, which leaves you a total of about 7 calories per spoonful better off.

––––––––––

THE POWER OF SPICES

Spices are a dieter's dream. They add bucketloads of flavour with zero additional calories and can transform a dull,
tasteless dish into one that is packed with flavour. Here are
some of the most frequently used spices that also contain
unexpected health benefits:

Turmeric The yellow pigment in turmeric, called curcumin, is known to contain potent antioxidant and anti-
inflammatory properties. Extracts of this spice may help
ward off heart attacks in people who have had recent
bypass surgery, so researchers have found.

Cinnamon Studies have shown this spice can inhibit the
growth of dangerous *E.coli* bacteria when added to foods.
It might also help lower blood sugar levels in people with
type-2 diabetes.

Ginger Daily ginger consumption has been shown to
reduce exercise-induced muscle pain by 25 per cent.

Chilli Some scientists have suggested that capsaicin, the
chemical that gives chilli pepper its fiery flavour, may help
to stave off obesity by cutting calorie intake, burning
energy and inhibiting the accumulation of body fat.

Cayenne Red cayenne pepper may help to curb the appetite and burn calories. One study found that about half
a teaspoon of cayenne pepper either mixed in food or

▶

swallowed in a capsule helped normal-weight young adults burn about 10 more calories over a four-hour period, and it also helped to decrease appetite.

Vegetables and fruit

By now we are all aware of the five-a-day mantra for healthy eating. This is based on advice from the World Health Organization, issued in 1990, which recommends eating a minimum of 400g (14oz) of fruit and vegetables a day to lower the risk of serious health problems, such as heart disease, stroke, type-2 diabetes and obesity. Research has proven that increasing fruit and vegetable consumption is the most important anti-cancer message after smoking, yet most of us still fail to meet the target.

The latest evidence from the European Food Information Council, based on a review of eating habits in 19 EU countries, showed that only four European countries met the WHO target: Poland (577g/1½lb), Italy (452g/1lb), Germany (442g/1lb) and Austria (413g/14½oz). Britons ate 258g (9oz) of fruit and vegetables a day, compared with the European average of 386g (13½oz). On average, UK men manage 4.1 portions a day, and women 4.8 portions. Swedish men and women are the worst fruit and vegetable consumers, with only 3.5 and 2.9 portions a day.

These findings are all the more concerning when you consider that many experts believe the five-a-day target is too low for fighting some killer diseases. Scientists at Oxford University analysed the lifestyles of more than 300,000 people across eight countries in Europe and found that people who ate at least eight portions of fruits and vegetables a day had a 22 per cent lower risk of dying from heart disease. Berries are a particularly rich source of antioxidants and plant compounds with many studies suggesting a high intake can have far-reaching health benefits. It helps that the sweetness of berries means we are more inclined to enjoy them and eat a bowlful without complaint.

This is one food group where more is generally better. What matters most when you select fruit and vegetables is variety and freshness. Choosing to try something different on a regular basis means a greater exposure to, and intake of, a range of vitamins and minerals. A good tip is to include as many different colours in your dish or on your plate as possible, as it is more likely that you will also be getting a diverse range of nutrients. Most fruits and vegetables are relatively low in calories, contain virtually no fat (with the odd exception) and are salt-free. What's to lose? Below are my top recommended vegetables, fruits and berries.

Top vegetable choices

Broccoli A rich source of immune-boosting vitamins C and K – important for blood clotting – broccoli also contains a nutrient called indole-3-carbinol that is thought to balance out oestrogen levels. Researchers at Oregon State University found that sulforaphane – a compound found in cruciferous vegetables, such as broccoli, pak choi and Brussels sprouts – has strong anti-cancer properties.

Sweet potatoes These vegetables get their orange colour from beta-carotene and are also an excellent source of vitamins C and E, which are important for skin health. US scientists compiled a table of 58 vegetables ranked according to their content of 7 important nutrients. Sweet potatoes scored 582 compared to the 114 scored by ordinary jacket potatoes. Sweet potatoes make a good choice and can be mashed, roasted or baked and served with a spoonful of low-fat fromage frais.

Carrots Rich in beta-carotene, the substance that gives carrots their orange colour, carrots are full of powerful antioxidants. Research shows that the anti-cancer properties of carrots are more potent if the vegetable is not cut up before cooking. Scientists found 'boiled before cut' carrots contained 25 per cent more of the anti-cancer compound falcarinol than those chopped first.

Kale has made something of a comeback as a super-food packed with antioxidants; sales of baby leaf kale, which is quicker to prepare and more tender to eat than the original curly kale, are soaring in supermarkets. The vegetable, which is a form of cabbage, has more calcium than broccoli and is high in vitamins A and C. It is also a good source of iron and contains plenty of vitamin K and the pigment lutein, which helps to promote eye health.

Beetroot is among the most widely studied of all vegetables in recent years. It contains nitrates, which have been shown to have a potent effect on sports performance. Other studies have shown beetroot can help to lower blood pressure, and it also contains anti-inflammatory properties in the form of acetylsalicylic acid, a relation to aspirin.

Top fruit choices

Nectarines Similar to peaches but with a smoother skin, nectarines are particularly rich in vitamin C – two fruits will give you a whole day's supply. Like other fruits and vegetables, they provide fibre, and the orange colour means it is a source of beta-carotene. Since a medium-sized nectarine only has 60 calories, they make a perfect mid-morning snack.

Plums Scientists found plums matched or exceeded blueberries – renowned for their health-giving properties – in the antioxidants and phytonutrients they contained, which help to prevent disease. Antioxidants are molecules that sweep through the body looking for health-threatening free radicals to knock out. One plum contains about the same amount of antioxidants as a handful of blueberries. Because plums are small (and juicy) it is easy to consume three or four in one sitting, but even that will add up to only 58 calories.

Apples With all the talk of 'super-foods', we tend not to consider apples worthy of such a grand title; however, according to a whole raft of new scientific research, which places apples at the top of the healthy-living tree, if you eat at least two apples daily you can reduce the risk of heart disease and other killers. Apples contain phytonutrients or phytochemicals (compounds found in plants), which act as antioxidants against LDL (low-density lipoproteins), the damaging portion of cholesterol in the bloodstream. They are also rich in the soluble fibres, pectins, which have been demonstrated to be effective in lowering cholesterol levels.

Cherries For a low-calorie nibble, cherries are hard to beat. A 400g (14oz) punnet contains only 108 calories. They are rich in D-glucaric acid, a super-nutrient said to help with lowering cholesterol. Eating about 20 a day provides between 12 and 25mg of anthocyanins, a compound that is a strong antioxidant and also has an anti-inflammatory painkilling effect; it has been shown to reduce the pain of gout. With an exceptionally low glycaemic index, cherries are great for stabilising blood sugar levels and keeping hunger at bay. They contain good levels of potassium, which regulates heart function and a cancer-fighting compound called ellegic acid.

Bananas Although they often get a bad rap for containing fewer nutrients than other fruits, bananas are a great source of potassium, and their high carbohydrate content makes them popular among sporty types as a between-exercise snack. It's a common misconception that ripe bananas contain more calories than unripe ones, but they do taste sweeter. The reason is that some of the starches present in the fruit are converted into sugars as the banana ripens. Calories don't increase, but sweetness does. It's worth opting for a slightly unripe banana if you can, as this will mean that it has a lower GI and therefore a greater level of sustained energy release. Because undigested starch passes into the large intestine, a less ripe banana actually means that fewer calories from it are absorbed.

Grapes are another fruit that are great for grazing. With only 300 calories per 500g (1lb 2oz) punnet, they are a good source of fibre (especially if they contain seeds). Black grapes contain resveratrol: a nutrient that is known to aid heart health. A University of Michigan Cardiovascular Center study suggested that grapes may prevent heart-health risks because of the phytochemicals – naturally occurring antioxidants – turning on a protective process in the genes that reduces damage to the heart muscle. In a trial, rats that ate a salty diet rich in black, green or red grapes had lower blood pressure, better heart function, and fewer signs of heart muscle damage than the rats that ate the same salty diet but didn't receive grapes.

Top berry choices

Blueberries The blueberry's countless health benefits are linked to its high content of flavonoids, a group of active substances that includes anthocyanin, the pigment that gives the berry its blue colour. Diets supplemented with blueberries have been shown to prevent memory loss and boost brainpower. They also contain resveratrol (see Grapes above), and recent studies have highlighted the cholesterol-fighting benefits of another blueberry antioxidant, pterostilbene.

Blackberries Although they contain less vitamin C than other berries – a 100g (3½oz) serving provides 15mg compared with 77mg in strawberries – they are still a useful source. Blackberries are also rich in anthocyanins, which are thought to have antibacterial properties. This is why the fruit is often recommended for sore throats. On the downside, these berries contain salicylate, a natural aspirin-like compound, which has been known to trigger a reaction in people who are allergic to aspirin.

Blackcurrants Weight for weight, blackcurrants contain four times as much vitamin C as an orange, making them one of the richest sources of the immune-boosting vitamin. One 15g (½oz) tablespoonful provides 30mg of the vitamin, three-quarters of the recommended 40mg daily intake. Blackcurrant skins contain the pigment anthocyanin, known to inhibit bacteria, including *E. coli* – a common cause of stomach problems and diarrhoea. Seeds of the blackcurrant contain gamma-linolenic acid, a high intake of which has been linked to the prevention of inflammatory diseases such as arthritis.

Strawberries Not only are strawberries an excellent source of vitamin C – they contain 77mg in a small, 100g (3½oz), bowl-ful, which is almost twice an adult's daily requirement – but they are also particularly low in calories, about 27 per 100g (3½oz), making them an ideal dieter's snack. Plant chemicals called p-coumaric acid and chlorogenic acid that are present in the fruit can help to prevent the formation of carcinogenic (cancer-forming) substances called nitrosamines in the stomach, thereby reducing the risk of cancer.

Bilberries are thought to improve eyesight. Studies into their effects on vision were prompted after pilots during World War II experienced improvement in their night vision after eating bilberry jam. Bilberries are not as rich in vitamin C as many berries – they contain 17mg per 100g (3½oz) – but are rich in disease-fighting antioxidant compounds like flavonoids and phenolic acids. Regular consumption of the fruit strengthens blood capillaries and reduces the tendency to bruise.

Salad leaves

Being high in water, all salad leaves contain zero fat and minimal calories, plus they contain valuable minerals and vitamins; however, their vitamin and mineral profile can be hugely different depending on the variety. Use the swaps below to find the most nutritious leaves for your low-calorie salad.

SWAP ▸ Iceberg

This crispy lettuce first made an appearance in the 1980s when it was considered a culinary breakthrough; however, it lacks taste, and with a very high water content provides little but crunch.

FOR ▶ Chicory

Chicory leaves make a great salad bowl addition, because they are packed with a form of soluble fibre called inulin, which helps to promote good bowel habits. It's also known to be a good prebiotic food (see page 98), enabling the gut to protect its healthy lining.

SWAP ▶ Green garden lettuce

Although a very fresh garden lettuce is hard to beat in terms of taste, it can become limp within a day or two, and most of the vitamin C it contains will disappear.

FOR ▶ Watercress

Rich in vitamin C – an average serving provides more than a quarter of the daily amount – this nutritional powerhouse has also been linked to cancer prevention. Scientists at Southampton University found that volunteers who ate 80g (2¾oz) of watercress a day – the equivalent of a single vegetable portion – had elevated levels of cancer-fighting molecules in their blood within hours of eating the salad leaves.

SWAP ▶ Romaine

Also called cos, this lettuce is long in shape with thick and firm leaves and a stiff central rib. The outer leaves are slightly bitter, but the ones in the centre are sweeter and more delicate. It's a great salad addition, but not the best nutrient provider. The mini version is called Little Gem.

FOR ▶ Spinach

Spinach leaves are packed with B vitamins, required for healthy nerves, antioxidants and lutein, a substance that helps to protect against age-related eye problems. Only use baby spinach leaves, not the larger leaves, in salads.

SWAP ▶ Oak leaf lettuce

There are several varieties of oak leaf lettuce – green, red and bronze – but all are essentially the same in terms of the nutrients they provide. Like most lettuces, it contains vitamin C, but others provide more.

FOR ▶ Lollo rosso

The characteristic red leaves on this lettuce are the result of the antioxidant-rich anthocyanidin pigments it contains. Research has shown that a high intake of such pigments can help to prevent blood clotting and the build up of cholesterol.

WHAT ABOUT BAGGED SALADS?

Bagged salads have become the healthy take on convenience food and we grab them as a quick alternative to vegetables and the time-consuming chopping of salad ingredients. Whether they are worth the considerable extra expense compared with fresh leaves is debatable though. Researchers at Cornell University reporting in the *British Journal of Nutrition* showed that a manufacturing

▶

technique used to keep the bagged greens crispy for longer also destroys vitamins and protective antioxidants. The process, called modified atmosphere packaging, is particularly damaging to vitamin C levels, one of the most common vitamins in salad leaves. Levels of the nutritious substances p-coumaric acid, caffeic acid and quercetin are also depleted in bags of salad, it was found. What's more, the shelf life of a pillow of lettuce leaves is extended using modified atmosphere packaging, which creates a balance of gases inside the bag to retain moisture and prevent browning. Old and torn leaves lose vitamin C more rapidly than a whole lettuce. Those that are labelled 'ready washed' are likely to have been doused in water containing chlorine, which can also affect nutrient levels. The verdict? Go for fresh, whole lettuce every time.

CHAPTER **FOUR**

▪

Dairy foods and eggs

PROTEIN-RICH DAIRY FOODS play an important role in many people's diet. They are a good source of calcium, which is vital in the promotion of a healthy skeleton, and they contain a range of vitamins and minerals. Despite their health profile, however, many dairy products are maligned for being high in fat – particularly saturated fat – and for causing intolerances and allergies.

Much of the evidence against saturated fat from animal sources is now being disputed (see page 25). It is now thought that some saturated fats from natural sources, such as many of those in dairy foods, may have health benefits rather than causing problems. It is the saturated fats in processed foods that occur as a result of chemical manufacturing techniques to 'harden' processed vegetable oils that are now linked to raised cholesterol levels and, in turn, to an increased risk of heart disease.

This chapter separates the good dairy foods from the bad and the downright ugly, guiding you towards sensible choices and dispelling some longstanding myths.

Milk

Billed as Mother Nature's most wholesome food in its purest form, milk contains good quantities of vitamins and minerals; it has no additives, artificial colourings or preservatives, and we have been weaned on the idea that it is nutritionally essential for our health. Although antibiotics and other drugs are routinely used in the dairy industry, researchers disagree about the quantities that are carried through to the milk that you buy and whether they pose a problem. If you want to enjoy milk that is free of these, opt for organic. A glass of the 'white stuff' provides a unique blend of protein, magnesium, potassium and B-vitamins, not to mention the calcium required to nourish thirsty bones.

Yet our consumption of milk has been falling for many years. Concerns about intolerances and that milk is 'fattening', coupled with health scares has seen the amount of cow's milk that is drunk in the UK fall from an average 96 litres (169 pints) per person to 82 litres (144 pints) in the last 12 years. Certainly, this is taking its toll in numerous ways. Two-thirds of teenage girls are deficient in iodine, which is a key nutrient for brain development in the womb. Studies have shown that the problem stems from the fact that schoolgirls are drinking less milk, which is a common source of iodine, with one glass providing about 50 per cent of daily iodine needs. Children with low iodine levels score lower in IQ tests, and even a mild iodine deficiency during pregnancy can cause mental impairment in children.

What's more, it is recommended by osteoporosis charities and the UK government that, in order to reach calcium needs, adults consume three portions of dairy a day; a 200ml (7fl oz/⅓ pint) glass of milk counts as one portion. There are other dairy sources of calcium – a 150g (5½oz) pot of yoghurt and a 30g (1oz) piece of cheese as well as non-dairy sources such as nuts, leafy green vegetables and tinned fish eaten with bones – but milk is the best dairy source and it also supplies a lot of other vitamins and minerals. A glass of milk, or milk on cereal, will provide a six-year-old child with over half their daily calcium intake. It also supplies vitamins A, C, D, E, K and the B-group vitamins, and also magnesium, zinc and potassium.

Whole milk is still a good choice for dieters

If you are trying to lose weight, switching to a lower-fat milk may be helpful. But even whole milk, at 134 calories per 200ml (7fl oz/⅓ pint) glass, is not as bad for the waistline as people think. A glass contains far fewer calories and less sugar than a chocolate bar and is much better for you. Many of the calories in milk come from its fat content. Whole milk is about 3.5 per cent fat; semi-skimmed milk contains 1.7 per cent fat; 1 per cent fat milk contains 1g of fat per 100ml (3½fl oz); and skimmed milk contains 0.3 per cent fat. These levels mean that cow's milk is not classed as a high-fat food. It's worth pointing out that while a switch to lower fat milk might mean fewer calories and fat, it also means fewer fat-soluble vitamins (A, D, E and K).

The changing views on milk

Why has milk attracted so much criticism? Central to the anti-milk argument are suggestions that it is swirling with natural cow hormones, including one called insulin-like growth factor I (IGF-1). These hormones are said to encourage cell growth and may help to spur prostate cancer and, to a lesser extent, ovarian and breast cancer although the debate about the issue is furious. There is evidence that organic milk may be worth the extra expense not only because cows that produce it graze in organic pastures and are not exposed to chemical farming agents such as the use of drugs and pasture fertilisers; findings published in the *Journal of Dairy Science* showed that organic supermarket milk contained higher levels of nutritionally beneficial fatty acids compared with 'ordinary' milk regardless of the time of year or weather conditions in which it was produced.

Much anti-milk sentiment is ill-founded; for example, dairy food, a major source of saturated fat, is a prime example of why scientists now suspect there is more to the fat story than was once thought (see Not all fat is the same, page 25). Research has proven that there's no direct link between milk and heart disease; on the contrary, findings suggest that the potassium in milk can help to lower blood pressure. Also, the fatty acid conjugated linoleic acid, found in milk, can help to reduce the risk of a heart attack.

In short, the negative evidence surrounding milk intake is inconclusive; for many of us milk remains the most bio-available and rich source of calcium in the human diet and in the West we consume relatively high amounts. This is not the case for many populations around the world, however, who are unable to digest the milk sugars; lactose intolerances are common in people of African and Asian descent, for example.

What's in a glass?

When it comes to fat and calorie content, there is a definite pecking order with milk. The most tasty milk, thanks to the fat globules that coat the tongue and tempt the palate as you drink it, is whole milk, although it is also the most calorific. Overall, even whole milk isn't particularly high in calories. It may be worth sticking to smaller quantities of whole milk if you don't want to sacrifice flavour, but otherwise, descend down the ladder in terms of fat content to make the greatest savings. Cow's milk doesn't contain enough iron for a young baby's needs and shouldn't be given until they are 12 months old when whole milk can be introduced into the diet. Semi-skimmed milk can be given from the age of two (provided your child is a good eater), but children under five should not be given skimmed or 1 per cent fat milk as neither contains sufficient calories to support a young child's calorie requirements for growth.

SWAP ▶ Whole cow's milk

Per 200ml (7fl oz/⅓ pint): calories 132; fat 7.8g

Packed with nutrients, including protein, calcium, zinc, and vitamins A and B, whole milk is often called a 'complete food'. Only tinned pilchards and sardines provide more calcium weight for weight than cow's milk, and osteoporosis charities recommend regular consumption of cow's milk to strengthen bones and provide some of the 800mg of the mineral needed every day for adults. This is the best kind of milk for children to drink because it contains the fat and vitamins needed for growth. If you want to reduce your calories though, swap it as below.

FOR ▸ Semi-skimmed milk

Per 200ml (7fl oz/⅓ pint): calories 100; fat 3.6g

The most popular type of milk sold in supermarkets, semi-skimmed contains about half the fat of whole milk and, as with other reduced-fat milks, slightly more protein and water-soluble vitamins. It is only suitable for children aged two years and above.

———

SWAP ▸ 1 per cent fat cow's milk

Per 200ml (7fl oz/⅓ pint): calories 80; fat 2.0g

This is the latest trend in milk consumption and it sits between skimmed and semi-skimmed milk. (Semi-skimmed milk contains 1.6 per cent fat and skimmed milk 0.1 per cent.) At some supermarkets, it has amassed a 10 per cent share of all milk sales, with people preferring its slightly richer taste to skimmed milk. It retains most of its nutrients including calcium but, because most of the fat is removed, the milk contains fewer fat-soluble vitamins. It is not recommended for children under five years, who need the fat in whole milk to aid growth and development.

FOR ▸ Skimmed milk

Per 200ml (7fl oz/⅓ pint): calories 70; fat 0.2g

The lowest fat content of milks available, skimmed milk contains slightly more calcium than whole milk but is not recommended for children under the age of five years, who need the extra energy and calories for essential growth. Since it is the fat in milk that adds flavour, the lower the fat content the more 'watery' milk can taste.

DRINK IT STRAIGHT FROM THE COW?

Raw, or unpasteurised milk, is sold in green-topped bottles and comes straight from the cow. Although it is widely touted as a cure-all for ailments ranging from psoriasis and high blood pressure to gut problems, tests on raw milk conducted by the UK government's Food Standards Agency have shown that it contains 'illness-causing pathogens' in the form of bacteria that could leave people prone to infection. Because of this, sales of the milk in the UK, which must carry a label warning of its risks, are restricted to farm shops in England and Wales. It has been banned in Scotland for over 25 years but is sold elsewhere and is gaining huge popularity in the USA and Canada.

Milk alternatives

Full-fat or skimmed milk were once the only choices available when it came to milk. Now chiller cabinets and shelves in supermarkets are heaving under the weight of cow's milk alternatives ranging from rice and buffalo milk to oat and sheep's milk.

For many people, cow's milk has become a dietary pariah, something to be avoided at all costs because the lactose, or milk sugar, contained therein triggers symptoms of bloating, constipation and abdominal pain. About ten million adults in the UK claim to have a food intolerance, and an inability to break down and absorb the sugar in cow's milk ranks among the most common. Whether or not everyone who believes they have a cow's milk intolerance actually has one is doubtful. One study involving 30 adults who described themselves as severely lactose intolerant found that 30 per cent of them were actually able to effectively absorb the milk sugar with no side effects. This means that almost one third of those who were cutting out dairy foods because they thought they had to in order to protect their health actually had no reason to avoid milk, yoghurt or cheese. Although some people might choose not to eat dairy foods, cutting dairy out because you think you have to can be complicated and confusing, as it is present in so many foods. Make sure you consult a state registered dietician who will confirm whether or not there is cause for concern.

Intolerances aren't the only reason people are making the switch to cow's milk alternatives. Others are cutting out cow's milk because of the belief that it is packed with hormones through intensive farming; however, although cow's milk can contain some natural hormones, British milk suppliers are not permitted to allow dairy cattle to ingest hormones. Also, as already discussed, people mistakenly fear that the fat content in milk will not help them to lose weight. As a result, sales of non-dairy milk alternatives have risen by one-fifth every year since the mid-1990s. But how do the vast array of cow's milk alternatives that are now available measure up?

It's worth pointing out that most milk alternatives are not suitable for children under 12 months of age.

SWAP ▶ Rice milk

Per 200ml (7fl oz/⅓ pint): calories 110; fat 2.4g

Popular among those who are soya and cow's milk intolerant, rice milk is made from filtered water, partially milled organic brown rice and sea salt. Commercial rice milk contains as much calcium and as many vitamins as cow's milk but less fat even than soya milk. It tastes sweeter than many milks and is low in calcium and protein.

FOR ▸ Oat milk

Per 200ml (7fl oz/⅓ pint): calories 70; fat 1.4g

A useful milk replacement for cooking and baking although it can also be drunk cold. Commercial oat milks are made from the liquid left when oats are soaked in water. Studies have shown that oats help to lower cholesterol levels and are a low glycaemic index food that provides a long-lasting energy burst. It is thought that the milk has similar benefits.

SWAP ▸ Buffalo milk

Per 200ml (7fl oz/⅓ pint): calories 220; fat 16g

With 11.5 per cent more protein than cow's milk, buffalo milk also has more of some vitamins and minerals, such as calcium and iron. Nutrition scientists are trying to modify the high protein content in buffalo milk into a protein similar to the one in human breast milk that reduces cancer. It also lacks the sour aftertaste of many cow's milk alternatives. But it does contain twice as much fat as whole cow's milk and is also high in calories.

FOR ▸ Sheep's milk

Per 200ml (7fl oz/⅓ pint): calories 198; fat 13.4g

Some people with an intolerance to cow's milk find sheep's milk a useful alternative, although many may find that they are unable to tolerate sheep's milk as well. Like goat's milk, it has small fat globules that are easily digested by the body. It contains up to twice as many minerals, such as calcium, phosphorus, zinc, and the important B-group vitamins, as cow's milk and is a rich source of iodine, an essential nutrient required for the synthesis of thyroid hormones. Note that it is not suitable for babies under a year old, as it doesn't have the correct balance of nutrients to meet a baby's needs.

———

SWAP ▶ Soya milk

Per 200ml (7fl oz/⅓ pint): calories 65; fat 4.8g

Soya milk is made from soaked, cooked and ground soya beans. When enriched, it provides the same levels of nutrients as cow's milk, including calcium, protein, potassium and vitamins A and D. It also contains a substance called genistein, which is thought to inhibit the formation of blood vessels that assist in the growth of small tumours, and some studies have linked a regular intake to a lower risk of breast, prostate and colorectal cancer. Soya consumption has also been linked to lower cholesterol and a reduced risk of heart disease. In their natural state, soya beans taste quite bitter, so the milk is heavily processed to mask the unpleasant flavour, which makes it less of a 'natural' alternative than many people think. Some varieties are highly sweetened, so check the label for hidden calories. Unsuitable for children under six months.

FOR ▶ Almond milk

Per 200ml (7fl oz/⅓ pint): calories 60; fat 2.2g

Good for vegans and lower in fat and calories than soya milk, this is a useful dairy milk alternative. It is made from ground almonds and can be used in cooking or as a drink. It contains no saturated fats or lactose (milk sugar) and is among the lowest in calories of all milk alternatives. In many commercial almond milks, almonds are the second or third ingredient after water and sweeteners, giving it a sweeter flavour than regular milk. Check the label to see whether it contains a lot of added sugar. Although nuts are a good source of protein and calcium, the levels in almond milk do not match those in soya, cow's or goat's milk.

———————

SWAP ▶ Goat's milk

Per 200ml (7fl oz/⅓ pint): calories 124; fat 7.8g

People with a mild intolerance to cow's milk might find goat's milk easier to digest, although it's often the case that there's a cross-over and those who struggle with cow's milk also have problems with goat's milk. It does contain similar levels of lactose (4.1 per cent compared with 4.7 per cent in cow's milk) so is not useful for those who are lactose intolerant. Some people believe the proteins form a softer curd in the stomach, which is alleged to aid diges-tion, although this hasn't been proven. Whole goat's milk has a slightly salty taste and is almost as high in calories and fat as whole cow's milk; semi-skimmed, lower fat versions are now available. It's unsuitable for children under one year old, as it doesn't have the right balance of nutrients to meet their needs. It also con-tains a substance that binds with vitamin B_{12} found in foods from animal sources to prevent the vitamin from being absorbed by the body; some children who have been given goat's milk have been found to have B_{12} deficiency, which can cause a type of anaemia, the symptoms of which are fatigue and weakness.

FOR ▶ Camel milk

Per 200ml (7fl oz/⅓ pint): calories 120; fat 5.8g

A newcomer to the alternative milk market, camel milk is lower in fat and calories than goat's milk, but contains five times as much vitamin C as cow's milk. Studies in India show that it contains high levels of insulin and is helpful to people with diabetes as it keeps blood sugar levels stable. In India it is also used therapeutically to treat a range of illnesses. It tastes watery and salty so is best used in cooking, although it can be used in other ways as well.

Cheese

With literally thousands of varieties of cheese on sale in super-markets, there is no denying that our love affair with this particular foodstuff endures. Often reviled by dieters for being one-third fat, there is more to cheese than meets the eye. As a general guide, harder cheeses such as Cheddar, Parmesan and Stilton contain the most fat (up to 35 per cent) whereas soft cheeses like Camembert and Brie contain less (about 26 per cent). Some very soft cheeses such as ricotta and cottage contain 12 per cent fat or less. The choice and variety is bewildering.

On the nutrition front, cheese is a valuable source of protein, which is vital for body tissue maintenance, and supplies 12 per cent of bone-building calcium in the diet. It contains vitamins B_2 (riboflavin), A and D and is a particularly good source of vitamin B_{12}, especially for those who don't eat meat.

There is plenty of evidence, too, that cheese may help to prevent tooth decay, due to its ability to stop tooth enamel being attacked by acids formed in the mouth when bacteria breaks food down. What seems to happen is that cheese stimulates the production and flow of alkaline saliva, which restores pH levels in the mouth. The proteins in cheese are also thought to coat and protect the enamel surface of teeth, preventing it from dissolving. All perfect reasons for that after-dinner serving of cheese and biscuits.

In supermarkets, most cheeses are given a strength rating of 1–5 (5 being the strongest flavour). There are factors other than taste to take into account when buying. Look out for salt content: blue cheeses, in particular, can contain more salt to balance out the other strong flavours. Others, such as feta and halloumi, are aged in salty brine, which bumps up their sodium count.

All values in the swaps section below are based on a 30g (1oz) serving of each cheese (a matchbox-sized piece).

SWAP ▶ Ricotta

Per 30g (1oz): calories 40; fat 3g; salt 0.6g

Lower in fat than many cheeses, crumbly ricotta is made from the watery whey left over when cow's milk is made into harder cheeses. Its calcium levels aren't great and although it is low in fat, calories and salt, there is an even more virtuous choice.

FOR ▶ Cottage

Per 30g (1oz): calories 19; fat 0.1g; salt 0.1g

As far as cheeses go, cottage provides the lowest you can get in terms of fat, calories and salt. It contains half the calories of even low-fat ricotta. The lack of creaminess means it doesn't have much flavour, but you can add your own with herbs such as fresh chives. It contains some calcium, but not a great deal – one-tenth the amount in Cheddar.

────────

SWAP ▶ Brie

Per 30g (1oz): calories 90; fat 7.5g; salt 0.5g

Although it has a reputation for being high in fat, Brie contains less fat and calories than Cheddar and Stilton. It is one of the best sources of calcium from among the softer cheeses, supplying 540mg per 100g (3½oz). Interestingly, the rind is a good source of vitamin B_1 (thiamine), essential for healthy nerves as well as for energy production. There are healthier options, however.

FOR ▶ Camembert

Per 30g (1oz): calories 85; fat 6.6g; salt 0.5g

As rich and creamy as it tastes, Camembert does in fact contain one-third less fat than Cheddar and even less than its creamy French counterpart, Brie. You also save 5 calories per serving with the switch. As with Brie, the rind contains vitamin B_1, so don't throw it away.

SWAP ▶ Stilton

Per 30g (1oz): calories 125; fat 10.6g; salt 0.6g

This English blue cheese is renowned for its strong flavour and smell. Unfortunately, it is also high in fat and has less than half the calcium content of Cheddar. Some varieties contain a lot more salt, so check the label.

FOR ▶ Gorgonzola

Per 30g (1oz): calories 92; fat 7.7g; salt 0.7g

A creamy blue alternative to Stilton, Gorgonzola saves you 33 calories and almost 3g of fat per serving if you eat it instead of Stilton. Like other blue cheeses it can be salty, so it's best served sprinkled into salads.

SWAP ▸ Goat's

Per 30g (1oz): calories 120; fat 9.6g; salt 0.5g

Made with goat's milk, this cheese has similar levels of calcium and vitamins to Cheddar. In a University of Granada study, researchers found that goat's milk (and cheese) contains a significant amount – and more than cow's milk – of oligosaccharides. These compounds reach the large intestine undigested and act like probiotics (see page 97), enhancing the growth of healthy probiotic gut flora, which wards off infections. But goat's cheese is not particularly low in fat or calories.

FOR ▸ Feta

Per 30g (1oz): calories 85; fat 6.9g; salt 0.9g

A Greek cheese made with sheep's milk, feta is low in calories, providing a 35 calorie saving per serving. By choosing feta you will also chop almost 3g of fat per matchbox-sized portion; however, feta has a high sodium content due to the fact that it is aged in salty brine. Consume 50g (1¾oz), which is not difficult to do even when it is served with a salad, and it gives you one-third of the recommended daily sodium intake for a woman.

––––––––

SWAP ▸ Soft cheese

Per 30g (1oz): calories 75; fat 7.2g; salt 0.3g

Soft creamy cheeses are as widely used in cooking and baking as they are for spreading on crackers and bread. Although they aren't the worst offenders in the calorie stakes, they contain a relatively low level of calcium (one-sixth of that found in Cheddar) and, unless you select the low-fat versions, they are not a dieter's dream.

FOR ▸ Quark

Per 30g (1oz): calories 22; fat 0.1g; salt negligible

What it lacks in flavour, quark more than makes up for in its low calorie and fat content. Use in place of creamy and soft cheeses in recipes that require them and you will save 53 calories per 30g (1oz).

———

SWAP ▸ Cheddar

Per 30g (1oz): calories 125; fat 10.5g; salt 0.6g

Cheddar is one of the best-selling but also the highest-fat cheeses around. On the upside it contains very useful amounts of calcium – 720mg per 100g (3½oz) – and some zinc, which is essential for the action of many of the enzymes in the body. Coloured and flavoured cheeses tend to add nothing nutritionally beneficial – indeed they can be sweetened and contain not just extra ingredients but additional calories as well. They are best avoided.

FOR ▸ Swiss Gruyère

Per 30g (1oz): calories 120; fat 9.6g; salt 0.5g

This is a semi-hard cheese with plenty of kick and is a good alternative to Cheddar. The calorie and fat saving isn't huge, but if you have two cheese sandwiches you will save about 10 calories and 2g of fat. Swiss Gruyère is also a very good source of calcium, providing 1,000mg per 100g (3½oz) serving.

———

SWAP ▶ Wensleydale

Per 30g (1oz): calories 115; fat 9.5g; salt 0.4g

A crumbly, mild semi-hard cheese that is not as high in calories as similar varieties such as Stilton and Cheddar, but neither is it a particularly low-fat choice.

FOR ▶ Edam

Per 30g (1oz): calories 80; fat 5.9g; salt 0.5g

With more calcium but fewer calories than many cheeses, Edam makes a good choice for a snack. Its salt content is relatively high, so it should be eaten sparingly if you have high blood pressure, but it's a better option than many others and saves 35 calories per 30g (1oz) serving when you substitute it for Wensleydale on your crackers.

SWAP ▶ Halloumi

Per 30g (1oz): calories 100; fat 7.8g; salt 0.9g

This traditional Greek cheese, often grilled or fried to be served, is soaked in brine during the ageing process, making it a salty choice. Reduced-fat versions are available but they tend to be rubbery and lack flavour.

FOR ▶ Mozzarella

Per 30g (1oz): calories 80; fat 6g; salt 0.2g

Traditionally made from buffalo milk, mozzarella is a medium-fat Italian cheese with a good calcium content and, even if it's not particularly low in calories, it saves you 20 calories and 1.8g fat per 30g (1oz) serving compared to halloumi. When heated, a little goes a long way.

Butter and spreads

For years, butter was considered the enemy of good health. Consume too much of it and you were asking for a heart attack – or so we were lead to believe. Far better, it was thought, to switch to spreads and margarines made not with highly saturated and artery-clogging animal fat but with plant oils that were rich in polyunsaturated fats that seemed to boost heart health rather than the reverse. Now, though, it is generally agreed that the argument is less clear cut.

What scientists have discovered is that the fats in margarine and spreads that we once thought to be superior in health terms may in fact be a risk factor for coronary heart disease and type-2 diabetes. What's behind this shift in thinking is the way that spreads are produced.

Margarines – far from natural

Most margarines and spreads are made from vegetable oils – the liquid oil being extracted from seeds or beans, neutralised, bleached, filtered and deodorised to render them tasteless and odourless.

In order to make the liquid oils more solid and spreadable, their structure needs to be modified. Until recently, the majority of spreads on sale underwent a process called hydrogenation, which is achieved by pumping hydrogen through the oil. Hydrogenation produces so-called trans-fats that have since been found to be more damaging than saturated animal fats and to raise blood cholesterol levels and clog arteries more significantly. Trans-fats are rife in many prepared meals and foods despite a swell of public and medical concern about their safety. Heart disease experts and scientists from the UK government's watchdog The National Institute for Health and Clinical Excellence (NICE) have called for the use of trans-fats to be reduced or banned as they already are in New York City and Denmark. Some spread manufacturers have adopted different procedures to make spreads and go to great lengths to ensure that their products can be labelled 'low in trans-fats'. One of the most widely used approaches now is 'interisification' which blasts fat molecules with enzymes or acids to change their structure. It is thought to be much safer than hydrogenation, but long-term studies may yet tell a different story. Trans-fats remain a menacing presence in foods we buy nevertheless. As yet, though, there are no regulations to make manufacturers and retailers mention trans-fats on ingredients labels, so how do you tell where they are lurking? Hydrogenated fats do have to be declared, so scan labels for hydrogenated vegetable oils (HVO) or fats and partially hydrogenated vegetable oil (PHVO) or fats.

Once chemically altered by one method or another, the vegetable oils are mixed with emulsifiers, which bind water and oil together, as well as colouring, flavouring, whey and brine. By law, the spreads must have vitamins A and D added to the same levels that you would find in butter. This sci-fi-sounding mixture is then blended, pasteurised and chilled before being served to you as a healthier choice in a well-labelled tub.

What some spreads do have in their favour is a lower fat content than butter; margarines contain the same amount of fat and calories as butter – about 73 calories and 8g of fat per small pat, enough for 1–2 rounds of toast. Check the label and you may find a spread that contains 53 calories and 5.9g of fat for the same serving size. But is it worth the switch? What matters when it comes to fat is your overall consumption (see page 30). My view – and that of a growing number of experts – is that it is better to eat sensible amounts of real butter than a scientific concoction that might save a few calories but about which we know precious little in terms of long-term health effects.

The non-dairy alternative

For those who can't eat dairy or who prefer not to buy butter, opt for one of the organic, non-hydrogenated olive oil spreads that are generally available in health foods shops.

The better butter

Butter is naturally rich in vitamins A and D as well as in selenium, which is found in the soil upon which the cattle are grazed and is important for protection against free-radical damage in the body and in the fight against cancer. Studies have suggested that organic butter may contain even higher levels of vitamins and minerals. And even the saturated fat it contains is not as harmful to health as previously thought (see Not all fat is the same, page 25). Some researchers have suggested that the naturally occurring nutrients in dairy foods, such as vitamin D and potassium, may offset the risks of saturated fat and protect against heart disease among those who eat them regularly but in moderation.

Of course, it's hard to beat butter when it comes to flavour. So the best choice here is surprising: switch from spreads to butter. Just make sure you don't overdo it.

Yoghurt

The original health food, yoghurt has been used since the 16th century for its healing properties and is promoted by naturopaths for its natural 'neutralising' benefits on the digestive system. It remains as popular today as ever. It is difficult to get a more natural food than plain yoghurt. Made by adding a bacterial culture to warm milk, a combination that releases lactic acid and produces the familiar and satisfying gloopy texture of yoghurt, it has been shown in studies to help in everything from lowering cholesterol and the risk of heart disease to easing diarrhoea and constipation.

Many of the therapeutic benefits come from the 'live' bacteria, such as the standard yoghurt cultures, *Lactobacillus bulgaricus* and *Streptococcus thermophilus*, that yoghurt contains. In recent years a swell of positive evidence relating to these so-called 'friendly bacteria' has lead to many manufacturers pushing their 'probiotic' products as superior in the 'live' bacteria stakes (see Probiotics – Are They Worth the Investment?, page 97). Labels stating that bio-cultures have been used mean that the yoghurts have been made using different bacteria – usually *Bifidobacteria* or *Lactobacillus acidophilus* – which have been shown in studies to have a more targeted health benefit, because they are the strains of bacteria naturally present in the human gut. Such yoghurts might offer slight advantages to those suffering from urinary or gastrointestinal problems, such as traveller's tummy or diarrhoea.

DID YOU KNOW?

Many people who are unable to tolerate cow's milk find they can digest yoghurt made with cow's milk without prob- lems. Why? When milk is made into yoghurt, the bacteria produce a substance called lactase, which breaks down the sugar in milk (lactose) that often triggers intolerance.

Which yoghurts are healthiest?

When perusing the maze of gut-friendly yoghurt-based prod- ucts and drinks, however, it's worth remembering that *all* yoghurts in the chiller cabinet have probiotic properties unless the product has been pasteurised. Evidence shows that even the standard yoghurt cultures can stimulate the production of friendly bacteria in the human gut and can help to maintain intestinal health. Only yoghurts labelled 'UHT' or 'long life' contain bacteria that is not 'live', because it has been killed off during the heat-treating manufacturing process. The message: be careful not to pay over the odds for something that is going to give you no additional health benefit over a cheap tub of natural yoghurt.

Nutritionally, there is plenty to shout about yoghurt. A 150ml (5fl oz/¼ pint) pot provides 40 per cent of an adult's daily calcium needs and 50 per cent of the daily requirement for phosphorous, also essential for maintaining a healthy skeleton. While manufacturers are keen to promote low-fat versions of yoghurts, even the whole milk variety is not going to break the calorie and fat bank. To be classed as low-fat in the UK, a food must contain no more than 3 per cent fat. Whole cow's milk yoghurt just tips over that mark, weighing in at 3.7 per cent fat, still well within a healthy range.

The hidden ingredients

What's more important to consider than the fat content is what else is added to the yoghurt you are buying. Those that appear to be the most nutritious because they are loaded with fruit and natural flavourings often contain large amounts of sugar. Some yoghurts are so far removed from the original version of the food that they really do not deserve to carry the label 'yoghurt' at all. By far the best option is to buy a plain yoghurt of your choice and throw in some fresh fruit or compote. That way you are guaranteed that it won't be overly sugary or contain any artificial sweeteners and colourings. If you do opt for ready-prepared versions, be careful what you choose.

For ease of comparison, the values in the swaps below are based on 100g (3½oz) of each yoghurt. Pot sizes vary from 100g (3½oz) to 175g (6oz) per individual serving, so be careful to check how much you will actually be consuming.

SWAP ▸ Muller corner crunch toffee hoops yoghurt

Per 100g (3½oz): calories 153; fat 5.5g; sugars 18.8g

This highly sugary dessert is no better for you than a chocolate bar and contains 11 per cent chocolate hoops as well as being highly sweetened. Since a pot is 135g (4¾oz) in size, you would actually guzzle back 206 calories in each serving. There are no health benefits in consuming it.

FOR ▸ Muller light toffee yoghurt

Per 100g (3½oz): calories 50; fat 0.1g; sugars 7.0g

If you really must indulge your sweet tooth, then this is a better option. It remains far from healthy, being packed with fructose, caramel syrup and sweeteners, but you do save a whopping 103 calories per 100g (3½oz) and over 5g of fat by choosing this rather than the toffee hoops variety.

———————

SWAP ▸ Natural plain yoghurt

Per 100g (3½oz): calories 124; fat 6.3g; sugars 9.8g

In many ways, natural plain yoghurt is the best choice you can make. It is far from a high-fat food, although the fat content (and taste) can vary according to the type of milk used; even when made with very creamy milk it provides only a 5 per cent fat content. Still, there are savings that can be made.

FOR ▸ Natural plain low-fat yoghurt

Per 100g (3½oz): calories 65; fat 1.6g; sugars 7.0g

Made with low-fat milk, this cuts calorie levels almost in half and reduces it to a low-fat food. Add fresh fruit and even a teaspoonful of honey for sweetness and you will be far better off than you would be buying some of the sugar-laden ready-made options.

———————

SWAP ▸ Natural Greek yoghurt

Per 100g (3½oz): calories 145; fat 11g; sugars 6.6g

It has a wonderful creamy consistency, but Greek yoghurt tends to be higher in fat than other varieties. Sometimes the whey that separates in the yoghurt is replaced with cream, which further bumps up the calories.

FOR ▶ Natural set yoghurt

Per 100g (3½oz): calories 71; fat 3.7g; sugars 5.5g

If it's a jelly-like consistency you're after in a yoghurt, then this is a lower fat and calorie choice. Often there is a watery liquid on top of the yoghurt, which is the whey in the milk that separates; it can be eaten or poured away. Flavoured set yoghurts contain no whole fruit so are best avoided.

SWAP ▶ Tesco finest strawberry and cream yoghurt

Per 100g (3½oz): calories 145; fat 7.7g; sugars 14.3g

Made with yoghurt and 13 per cent whipping cream and sweetened with sugar, the redeeming feature in this strawberry and cream yoghurt is that it contains 18 per cent strawberries; however, the fruit content does nothing to alter the fact that this product is 24 per cent sugar and 17 per cent fat. Because the pot size is 150g (5½oz), you would actually be consuming 215 calories per serving.

FOR ▶ Danone activia 0 per cent fat strawberry yoghurt

Per 100g (3½oz): calories 60; fat 0.1g; sugars 9.7g

Although not exactly a yoghurt in its most natural state (it contains stabilisers, flavouring, colouring and artificial sweeteners, not to mention fairly high amounts of sugars), this does at least offer considerable savings on fat and sugar as well as calories compared with the Tesco yoghurt. It contains bio cultures and 9 per cent strawberries.

SWAP ▶ Sainsbury's lemon curd yoghurt

Per 100g (3½oz): calories 162; fat 6.7g; sugars 21.1g

This mix of sugar (the most prominent ingredient), whipping cream, egg and butter is sweeter than some desserts. It contains only 4 per cent lemon juice and a tiny amount of lemon pulp and oil.

FOR ▶ Rachel's organic coconut yoghurt

Per 100g (3½oz): calories 156; fat 11.1g; sugars 10.1g

Switch to this product and you save 24 calories per 100g despite the fact that it contains cream and some sugar. The only other ingredients are organic coconut (5 per cent) and organic yoghurt – an impressively short list in this marketplace. Granted, the fat levels place it in the medium range, but it is still worth the switch.

SWAP ▶ Yeo Valley Greek honey yoghurt

Per 100g (3½oz): calories 148; fat 8.1g; sugars 14.3g

This is made with organic yoghurt and sweetened with 6 per cent organic honey, which pushes its sugar content very close to a high level. As with milk, there is some evidence that opting for organic yoghurt may offer nutritional benefits. Scientists have shown that organic cow's milk, from which organic yoghurts are made, contains more fat-soluble nutrients. In this case, however, the downfall is the sugar and calorie content.

FOR ▶ Rachel's organic low-fat rhubarb yoghurt

Per 100g (3½oz): calories 84; fat 1.6g; sugars 13.3g

Containing only three ingredients – low-fat yoghurt, organic rhubarb (9.5 per cent) and some sugar – this is among the more natural choices of the vast array of yoghurts on sale. Generally, the fewer ingredients on a list the better. What's more, you will save 64 calories and 6.5g of fat by opting for this over the full-fat honey yoghurt.

ARE PROBIOTICS WORTH THE INVESTMENT?

Over the last two decades, it might have seemed our guts had never had it so good. With the rapid growth in probiotic products that claim to replenish the gut-friendly bugs that are said to ward off digestion problems and disease, many of us now swallow the promise of improved digestive health with these products. Available as drinks, yoghurts, powders and capsules, we currently spend millions on probiotics all in the hope of keeping harmful bacteria at bay. But is it money well invested?

Certainly, a growing number of manufacturers have jumped on the probiotic bandwagon, discovering and patenting their own particular beneficial bacteria that, they claim, has specific health benefits. But the jury is still out on whether they really are as potent as many believe. For all the positive studies that suggest probiotics are helpful to people with problems, ranging from irritable bowel syndrome to allergies, there are now many negative studies that throw their effectiveness into doubt.

The problems with probiotic foods and supplements

There are several areas of concern. For starters, only highly resistant forms of bacteria such as *Lactobacillus* and *Bifidobacteria* have been shown to survive transit to the gut; others are likely to be destroyed by the highly acidic environment in the stomach. If taken as a supplement, unless the capsules have a special enteric coating, they won't survive the transit through the stomach to reach the gut. There is also the issue that heat destroys probiotic bacteria, so if you take a cup of coffee just before or after consuming probiotic products, the beneficial bacteria will be killed off.

It is important to check the label on probiotic foods, too, as many products that appear to be healthy because they are loaded with probiotics are also loaded with sugar, which offsets any benefits the beneficial bacteria might have.

Lax labelling laws also mean that it is difficult for people to know which products are likely to be effective. One study found that 50 per cent of probiotic products on the market do not have the levels of healthy bacteria claimed on the label. Shoppers should be suspicious unless manufactures stipulate that a capsule or drink provides a minimum of ten million bacteria per dose. One probiotic powder was withdrawn from sale after it was shown to contain raised levels of *Clostridium difficile*, a bacteria that causes diarrhoea and colitis.

The essential role of prebiotics

If our guts are suffering from the strain of modern living, how do we keep them in check? It is now thought that the

▶

new good guys on the block – prebiotics, which are naturally present in food and easily obtained in the diet – are what we should have been taking all along. Whereas probiotics provide new doses of bacteria, prebiotics nourish and feed the friendly bacteria that is already present in the gut. Found naturally in breast milk, prebiotics are also present in foods that contain non-digestive carbohydrate substances, such as inulin, which sail through the digestive system and are fermented to boost the immune system. Foods high in inulin include dandelion leaves (added to a salad), Jerusalem artichokes, oats, chicory, bananas, garlic and onions. Some types of honey have prebiotic properties, thanks to the complex sugars, or oligosaccharides, they contain. Scientists at the Institute of Food Research in Norwich identified potential prebiotic properties in almonds that had been finely ground, which significantly increased the levels of certain beneficial gut bacteria when added to the diet.

Consume as many naturally occurring prebiotics as possible, by eating plenty of fresh fruit and vegetables, as these all help to keep your gut bacteria healthy.

Eggs

The ultimate convenience food, eggs are firmly back in fashion with sales up 10 per cent since 2000. Part of the reason for this increased popularity is the emerging evidence that eggs eaten in moderation are not a risk to heart health as was once thought and are actually good for us.

Not long ago, recommended egg consumption was limited to three per week to avoid a rise in blood cholesterol levels, but government advisors now put no upper limit on the number of eggs you can eat in a week as long as they form part of a healthy, balanced diet. Eggs received an undeservedly bad name because it was wrongly assumed by government health advisors and some researchers that the cholesterol contained in the yolks would raise blood cholesterol levels. That is now known not to be the case. Blood cholesterol levels are raised by a diet high in the trans-fats often found in pastry, processed meats, biscuits and cakes, and by some forms of saturated fat, such as palmitic acid, but not by the cholesterol in food.

Much of the proof that eggs are not a harmful addition to the diet hailed from the University of Surrey's school of biomedical and molecular science where a review of 30 egg studies carried out over 30 years revealed that they have no 'clinically significant impact' on heart disease or cholesterol levels. Researchers at Harvard University showed that people consuming one or more eggs a day were at no more risk of cardiovascular disease than non-egg eaters.

The healthy benefits

In fact, eating two eggs a day might help people to cut cholesterol levels, not raise them. To test this, a group of overweight but otherwise healthy volunteers were asked to eat two eggs a day for 12 weeks while they simultaneously followed a reduced-calorie diet prescribed by healthy-heart charities, while a control group followed the same diet but cut out eggs altogether. Both groups experienced a drop in the average level of blood cholesterol and also lost between 3kg (6lb 8oz) and 4kg (8lb 13oz) in weight.

There's other good news. Eggs are a good source of vitamins and minerals. Each yolk provides 13 essential nutrients
(egg whites contain albumen, which is an important source of
protein, but contains no fat) including the B-vitamin group,
which is needed for vital functions in the body, and also provides good quantities of vitamin A, essential for normal growth
and development.

Despite the fact that they are not exceptionally low in
calories – a large egg contains 75 calories and 5g of fat – they
might help with weight loss. When overweight women were
given either an egg or bagel breakfast, each providing the
same number of calories, the women eating the eggs felt fuller,
were less inclined to snack on fatty foods and consumed fewer
calories overall in the following 24 hours. The researchers
concluded that it was the protein in eggs that contributed to
satiety, suggesting a carbohydrate-only breakfast (such as bagels
or toast) would be unfulfilling.

Since eggs are a positive addition to the diet, this section
contains no swaps. Instead, there are recommendations on how
best to prepare and eat them for optimum health benefits.

GOOD WAYS TO COOK EGGS

Cooking eggs has very little effect on their nutrient content; however, it is best to prepare them using methods
that require the addition of no extra fat. Poaching or boiling eggs are the healthiest ways of cooking them. Scram-
bling with milk is fine, but adding cream will bump up
calories and fat, as will frying eggs. Scrambled eggs made
with butter and cream can contain as many as 316 calories
per serving.

Egg facts

The nutrients found in egg yolks, called lutein and zeaxanthin, could help to prevent or even reverse the age-related eye problem macular degeneration (MD). MD is one of the leading causes of blindness in the Western world, which occurs naturally as a consequence of getting older, although low lutein intake is implicated as a risk factor. Volunteers ate either cooked spinach, eggs or one of two types of lutein supplement, each providing 6mg of lutein per day. Those subjects who ate eggs had blood lutein levels three times greater than those who consumed it from the other sources.

Brown or white? Both shell colours for eggs are good. Although brown eggs are often considered healthier, there is no difference in taste or nutrition between different-coloured eggs. Indeed, whereas British consumers prefer brown eggs, US consumers buy more white. The difference? White-shelled eggs are produced by hens with white feathers and ear lobes; brown-shelled eggs are generally produced by hens with brown feathers and red ear lobes.

Storing eggs correctly is vital to maintaining their freshness and nutrient content. Ideally, buy fresh eggs or those from a reputable retailer who will have ensured they have been transported and stored at the correct temperature (below 20°C/68°F), then store the eggs, in their box, in a cool place once you get them home. Store eggs separately from other foods and make sure you use eggs by the 'best before' date shown on the egg or box.

Which eggs should you buy?

Perhaps more than any other foodstuff, the labelling and terminology used to sell and promote eggs is a minefield. In the egg department of a UK supermarket, it is not unusual to come across half a dozen or more terms used to describe what is, essentially, the simplest and most natural of foods. You can select from 'farm fresh', 'free-range', 'farm-assured' and 'freedom' eggs to 'barn-raised', 'corn-fed' and organic. All sound appealing in their own way, so which one to choose? Thankfully, eggs sold through supermarkets and shops (other than farm shops) in the UK are required to use a coding stamp, and this is the most reliable indicator of how they have been produced. Ignore flowery terminology, which often has no real meaning; for example, the term 'freedom eggs' is the RSPCA's own labelling scheme and it does not necessarily mean that they are free range. Check for the following instead:

Organic eggs Produced by birds that have a minimum of 10 square metres (33 square feet) of roaming space and with constant access to certified organic outdoor space during the daytime. Flock sizes are relatively small and no antibiotics are used in the feed.

Free-range eggs Produced by un-caged birds that are housed in sheds and lay naturally in nests. They have constant daytime access to outdoor space and a minimum of 4 square metres (13 square feet) space in which to roam.

Barn eggs Produced by birds that are kept indoors, albeit in large sheds with some space to roam and fly around naturally.

Battery eggs The least desirable option, although the EU has introduced new laws surrounding battery-egg production, which means that they have slightly more space and nest boxes, which is an improvement on conditions pre-2012. Hens used to be housed four to a cage with little space to move naturally and were required to produce 300 eggs a year. Due to raised awareness of the intensive production of battery eggs, our consumption of them has dropped from 85 per cent of all eggs consumed to under 60 per cent.

CHAPTER **FIVE**

.

Breakfast

THERE IS MUCH TRUTH in the saying that to 'breakfast like a king' is a route to wellness. Indeed, researchers have proven that kicking off the day by eating a hearty meal can help to keep you feeling full until lunchtime, warding off hunger pangs that might otherwise lead to high-fat snacking. Breakfast-eaters have been shown to be slimmer than breakfast-avoiders, and they have also been found to perform better in tests of mental agility and to have a boosted metabolism that burns energy more efficiently.

There are other advantages. It is now known that mental capacity or intelligence is not dependent on your brain's size, nor on the number of brain cells, or neurones, it contains. It is your brain's ability to make fast connections between the neurones that counts. The quicker those connections, the more information you can process. And eating the right foods, especially for breakfast, has been shown to enhance those neurone connections. In short, eat the right breakfast and you give yourself a head start when it comes to staying on top of what the day ahead throws at you; skip it and you will be forever playing catch-up.

Not all breakfast favourites are healthy. Our lifestyles dictate that we don't always have time to sit down and enjoy our first meal of the day at leisure, and so more of us grab breakfast on the run. Sales of takeaway breakfast snacks from coffee shops and fast-food restaurants have soared in recent years. That morning croissant, breakfast bar or breakfast panini is certainly convenient, but is it healthy? More often than not, the answer is a resounding 'No' and, in recent years, the nutritional profile of our most important meal of the day has been steadily declining.

As healthy as they look, breakfast cereals are among the worst offenders. Surely the wholesome and satisfying crunch served with cold milk is guaranteed to get you off to a high-energy start? Unfortunately, that is not always the case. What looks healthy on the packet is not always as nutritious inside. Too many of the most popular cereals available are so high in sugar, salt and fat that they are no better for you than a burger and chips or a bowlful of sticky toffee pudding topped with clotted cream. And although manufacturers have taken steps to reduce the sugar and salt content of their products, aiming to bring them into line with healthy-eating recommendations, many still contain 0.5g or more of salt per serving – the same as in some packets of crisps.

What's more, some varieties contain more sugar in a bowl than you would find in a bar of chocolate or a jam doughnut. Eat sugary breakfasts every day and the consequences for your long-term health are far from favourable. A high sugar intake is linked to obesity, diabetes, heart disease, cancer and liver problems. It triggers unwelcome shifts in metabolism and hormone levels and increases blood pressure levels. No surprises, then, that scientists have shown that excessively sugary diets contribute to 35 million deaths a year worldwide.

So how should you start your day? What will give you the optimal energy boost instead of overloading your system with sugar and fat? Almost certainly, the best breakfasts are the simplest in terms of the ingredients they contain, the sort of thing you can rustle up at home, adding your own touch when it comes to flavourings. But the next few pages will tell you everything you need to know about starting the day well.

GO FOR A POWERHOUSE BREAKFAST

What propels many elite athletes to top endurance performances? A protein powder? A super-energy drink? No – a bowl of porridge. For endurance activities such as distance running, a pre-race breakfast has been shown by sports scientists to be the most important meal. And porridge oats offer more of a boost than high-tech sports drinks and energy bars when it comes to prolonging energy levels and burning fat. It is the low glycaemic index (or GI) of porridge that makes it such a fitness-friendly fuel: low to moderate GI foods trigger the body to burn fat more quickly so that it can be used to fuel the muscles, thereby conserving carbohydrate (stored in the body as glycogen) to be used later. As a result, you can keep going for longer.

Remember, too, that an egg is a great way to start the day, see Good Ways to Cook Eggs on page 101 and Hot Breakfast Favourites starting on page 123.

Breakfast biscuits and bars

Eating a breakfast biscuit or bar seems to be a solution for breakfast on the go. They are hugely popular in parts of Europe and the market for such products in the UK is starting to boom. In most cases, however, the bars fail to live up to their claims of being an adequate substitute for a wholesome morning meal. Many are little more than glorified biscuits: overly processed and high in refined sugars. As an occasional stop-gap, though, they are better than eating nothing – provided you select carefully.

All values below are per bar or serving:

SWAP ▸ Belvita breakfast muesli biscuits

Per 4 biscuit serving: calories 228; fat 8.0g; sugars 12.0g; salt trace

The manufacturers make much of a clinical trial that showed that when these biscuits are eaten with fruit and dairy, such as a glass of milk, they regularly release carbohydrates over four hours to provide long-lasting energy and keep you full all morning. But a serving of Belvita (four biscuits) is high in sugars and medium-high for fat. You'd have a far better energy boost from a wholegrain cereal.

FOR ▸ Food Doctor pineapple and banana bar

Per 35g (1¼oz) bar: calories 107; fat 1.2g; sugars 8.4g; salt trace

This is a much more substantial bar. With well over one-third (35 per cent) of its content comprising dried banana and pineapple, it provides one-sixth of the daily target for fibre, which means it will be more filling than a highly processed biscuit-type bar and is very low in fat. And it saves 121 calories compared to the Belvita biscuits.

SWAP ▶ Dorset Cereals honey granola bar

Per 40g (1½oz) bar: calories 193; fat 11.4g; sugars 9.2g; salt trace

The redeeming feature of this bar is that it is free from additives. But it does contain oil and is sweetened with honey, sugar and agave nectar, a substance that raises blood sugar levels less rapidly than sugar but has little effect here as the bar contains both. It is a high-fat and high-sugar food.

FOR ▶ Nakd berry delight

Per 35g (1¼oz) bar: calories 135; fat 5g; sugars 16g; salt trace

Basically the berry delight is a dried-fruit bar with the only sugar it contains having occurred naturally in the dates (49 per cent), raisins (17 per cent) and raspberries (3 per cent). With cashew nuts also included, it contains an impressive 6 per cent fibre, one-quarter of the GDA for adults. It also contains 58 fewer calories and saves you 6g of fat.

SWAP ▶ Kellogg's elevenses cherry oat bakes

Per 50g (1¾oz) bar: calories 207; fat 8g; sugars 17g; salt trace

What is described as 'a bar that is packed full of whole oats and mixed with delicious ingredients' is, in fact, a cake designed to be eaten as a late breakfast snack. Granted, one-third of its content is oats, but they are mixed with oil, sugar syrup, glucose syrup, sweetened dried fruit, sugar and golden syrup to make a high-sugar food with almost one-fifth of your daily sugar limit in a couple of mouthfuls.

FOR ▸ Weetabix oaty strawberry bar

Per 23g (1oz) bar: calories 69; fat 1.4g; sugars 4.2g; salt trace

A small, oat-based cereal bar that is unlikely to stave off hunger pangs for long. It is, however, a preferable option than some of the chocolate-covered, sugar-loaded rivals on the market such as the cherry oat bakes, and will slice off 138 calories. The fruit content is low – only 7 per cent of the bar's weight is from dried strawberry pieces – but it is low in fat. Eat with some fresh fruit or yoghurt to ward off a grumbling stomach.

––––––––––

SWAP ▸ Trek peanut and oat bar

Per 68g (2¼oz) bar: calories 239; fat 8g; sugars 26g; salt trace

At more than double the size (or triple in some cases) of many other bars and with no added sugar, this 62 per cent dried fruit-and-nut-laden product will probably tide you over for longer than most. Fat comes from some added peanut butter, and apple juice boosts sweetness, but it is very high in sugars.

FOR ▸ Jordans frusli juicy raisins and hazelnuts

Per 30g (1oz) bar: calories 117; fat 3.7g; sugars 9.6g; salt trace

This bar contains 38 per cent dried fruit and nuts combined with oat flakes. You would think that would be sufficient to make it naturally sweet, so why add not only glucose syrup but also sugar and honey, resulting in a huge 32 per cent sugars content? Its redeeming feature is that it is lower in calories and fat than many bars and still contains 16g of sugar less than the Trek bar.

Breakfast cereals

What's in your breakfast cereal is not always easy to determine. On labels detailing nutritional value, manufacturers often use serving sizes of 30g (1oz) which falls far short of the amount the average person pours into their bowl (see also Check the Label, page 40). Many cereals contain high levels of sugar and salt, and are best avoided.

By far the best choices are those with minimal items listed in their ingredients panel, such as weetabix and shredded wheat. Porridge tops the lot (see Children's Breakfast Cereals on page 217), and the good news is that we like it. We get through 47 million gallons of porridge every year, with sales among the 24 to 35-year-old market rising by 80 per cent now that more is known about the health benefits of porridge. Studies have shown that a regular consumption of oats can help the body to hoover up cholesterol, fend off heart disease, suppress the appetite and beat depression. A study of almost 400,000 men and women found that those who ate lots of fibre-rich foods cut their risk of dying prematurely by a fifth. And with its long-lasting energy boost (porridge has the power to keep you going for precisely 4 hours and 21 minutes) it lessens the likelihood of snacking before lunch. All very good news for the waistline.

What else constitutes a good swap? All of the following values are based on a more realistic 50g (1¾oz) serving, unless otherwise stated (although that still falls short of the mark for many people). Remember to add calories and fat from the milk you pour over your cereal. An average serving of 150ml (5fl oz/¼ pint) of semi-skimmed milk will provide 75 calories and 2.6g of fat while the same amount of whole milk provides 99 calories and 5.25g of fat.

SWAP ▶ Bran flakes with dried fruit

Per 50g (1¾oz) serving: calories 190; fat 3.0g; sugars 12.0g; salt 0.5g

This healthy-looking combination of wholemeal bran flakes with dried fruit is high in fibre (providing 4g per bowlful) but also high in sugar, partly because of the dried fruit and partly because of the sugar added to make the flakes. If you are an adult trying to lose weight, then this is not the most sensible option.

FOR ▶ Shredded wheat

Per 45g (1½oz) serving (2 biscuits): calories 153; fat 1.1g; sugars 0.4g; salt trace

Since the only ingredient in this product is wholegrain wheat, it is naturally low in sugar, salt and fat, and is among the few commercial cereals to be classified as healthy for both salt and sugar. In fact, with 0.7 per cent sugar, shredded wheat has one of the lowest sugar counts of all commercial cereals. It is also a good source of fibre with two biscuits providing almost one-quarter of the guideline daily amount. Swap a bowl of fruit bran flakes for 2 shredded wheat and you save 37 calories. Top with fresh fruit for a dose of vitamin C and fibre.

———

SWAP ▸ Kellogg's crunchy nut

Per 50g (1¾oz) serving: calories 201; fat 2.5g; sugars 17.5g; salt 0.4g;

Cornflakes dipped in honey and roasted nuts sounds so healthy but provides a shockingly high 35 per cent sugar. It's hardly surprising when you scan the ingredients label and find that the cereal is sweetened with brown sugar, white sugar and honey.

FOR ▸ Cornflakes

Per 50g (1¾oz) serving: calories 189; fat 0.45g; sugars 0.6g; salt 0.5g;

Cornflakes aren't the best cereal option, as they are highly processed and offer little in the way of fibre, but they are preferable to many of the very highly sweetened brands. Be aware that the salt content is fairly high. Still, you will shave off some calories and save almost 17g of sugar per bowlful by swapping to these.

SPRINKLE ALMONDS ON YOUR CEREAL

People who eat a breakfast containing whole almonds felt full for longer and recorded lower concentrations of blood glucose after breakfast and lunch than people who did not have the nuts, a study in the *Journal of Nutrition and Metabolism* found. Almonds are low on the glycaemic index, which measures how quickly they cause blood sugar levels to rise after eating. Whereas foods that are quickly digested cause blood sugar to spike and then plummet, low-GI foods, such as almonds, cause a slower rise in blood sugar, which leaves people feeling fuller for longer.

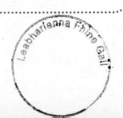

SWAP ▶ Alpen original

Per 50g (1¾oz) serving: calories 188; fat 2.9g; sugars 11.5g;
salt 0.14g

Alpen original is a sweetened muesli containing almost 25 per
cent added sugar and bulked up with milk whey powder and
dried skimmed milk, which gives it a powdery consistency. Its
fruit and nut content (total 14.5 per cent) is low compared to
many brands and, on the nutritional and particularly the fibre
front, you are far better off either making your own or selecting
a non-sweetened variety.

FOR ▶ Kellogg's all bran

Per 50g (1¾oz) serving: calories 167; fat 1.75g; sugars 9g;
salt 0.2g

This is sweetened with sugar, but contains less than Alpen and
is also lower in calories by a small margin. Serve with some fresh
fruit to boost your vitamin C intake.

———

SWAP ▶ Quaker oat granola

Per 50g (1¾oz) serving: calories 210; fat 4.75g; sugars 11.5g;
salt trace

Granola – oats that are toasted in oil and often sweetened –
seems a healthy option, but beware: varieties such as this
can contain more sugar per bowlful than a can of fizzy drink,
and they are also high in fat. Granola with fruit added means
more fibre, but this is not a good example of a wholesome
breakfast, with sugar and glucose syrup making it very sweet.

FOR ▶ Dorset Cereals fruits, nuts and seeds muesli

Per 50g (1¾oz) serving: calories 189; fat 5.7g; sugars 12.1g; salt trace

The energy in this unsweetened muesli comes from the fruit, nuts and seeds rather than added sugar. In fact, almost one-third of the weight of this product comes from the raisins, apricots, sultanas, dried banana, sunflower and pumpkin seeds, and nuts that provide valuable fibre and a range of nutrients including iron and potassium. A far more wholesome start to the day and you save 21 calories.

MAKE YOUR OWN MUESLI

Prepare your own muesli with oats, dried fruit, nuts and grains, such as barley and rye flakes, to ensure that you have the healthiest ingredients available. Bircher muesli is a variation that is incredibly easy to make: soak oats in fruit juice or milk overnight and add grated apple, toasted nuts and fresh berries for a wholesome start to the day.

BE WARY OF CLAIMS

Ignore claims that cereals 'supply energy' or are 'highly nutritious' – they are meaningless. Another term to over-look is the 'low in fat' label. Cereals are naturally low in fat, most containing about 3 per cent or less, and any that have fat added (like highly processed crunchy, granola-type cereals) are best avoided.

Fry-up, anyone?

A traditional fry-up might seem like the unhealthiest option on the morning menu, but surprisingly there are far worse offenders; however, it should remain an occasional treat, because 2 rashers of bacon, 1 sausage, 1 fried egg, baked beans, 1 slice of white toast, mushrooms and 1 grilled tomato provides 540 calories and 26.2g of fat. A white chocolate and strawberry muffin and a large latte with whole milk, on the other hand, provides a colossal 843 calories and 45.3g of fat with far less fibre and fewer vitamins.

Another traditional favourite, the bacon sandwich, might boost brain performance, one team of scientists suggested. In a study of 50 children, those who were given a bacon sandwich and a glass of fruit juice for breakfast performed better in verbal and non-verbal tests than children given cornflakes or toast and orange juice. It seems the protein in foods such as bacon, combined with the vitamins in fruit juice provide mental stimulation. Its fat and salt profile and the damaging nitrates present in many types of bacon, however, means a bacon sarnie shouldn't be too regular a treat. One review of evidence by the Harvard School of Public Health showed that a daily serving of 50g of cured or processed meat such as bacon (that's the equivalent of two rashers) could raise the risk of both heart disease and type-2 diabetes. What is more, as healthy as it might seem, too much fruit juice isn't a great breakfast addition, because it causes blood sugar levels to spike.

Breakfast muffins and pastries

What could look and smell more appetising than a freshly baked croissant? Or what could seem more nutritious than a muffin bursting with blueberries? Increasingly, pastries and muffins are the breakfast of choice for those who grab their morning snack at a coffee shop or café on the way to work. Unfortunately, these seemingly innocent breakfast choices can provide far more than you bargained on getting with your coffee.

All the values below are based on serving sizes sold in large coffee shop chains, but as serving sizes vary you need to remain hawk-eyed to check that the particular product you are buying doesn't contain more sugar and fat. As you will see, you need to select carefully to make sure you don't consume the equivalent of sticky toffee pudding every day.

SWAP ▶ Pain au raisin

Per shop-sized serving: calories 432; fat 20.8g; sugars 20.5g; salt 0.7g

Pastry made with butter and a crème pâtissière filling provide the whopping fat content of this breakfast snack – almost one-third of a woman's recommended daily intake. With about 12g it also provides more than half of the upper limit of saturated fat you should get in a day and it is also laden with sugars. And, despite the raisins it contains, it is low in fibre.

FOR ▶ Butter croissant

Per shop-sized serving: calories 304; fat 15.9g; sugars 5.0g; salt 0.6g

Save 128 calories by swapping to a plain croissant with no filling. Remember though, that plain croissants are best eaten alone, as you can add about 50 more calories for a small pot of jam.

————

SWAP ▶ Blueberry muffin

Per shop-sized serving: calories 430; fat 22.6g; sugars 26.2g; salt 0.7g

What appears to be a nutritious start to the day that is bursting with fruit is, in fact, about as healthy as eating a large slice of fudge cake and cream for breakfast. Containing almost one-third of the day's recommended sugar and fat intakes and almost one-quarter of a woman's daily calories, it is also low in fibre with the blueberries doing little to boost its nutritional profile. Avoid it if you are watching your waistline.

FOR ▶ Fruit scone

Per shop-sized serving: calories 337; fat 10.9g; sugars 23.3g; salt 1.2g

Despite being high in sugar, a fruit scone is one of the better choices in terms of fat as it contains half the amount in some pastries and muffins, the blueberry version included. Be careful not to add too much extra butter or jam, which would bump up the sugar and fat count even more. If you can find a wholemeal scone (although they are not widely available in coffee chains), you would get more fibre. A downside is the salt content: it contains more than a rasher of bacon (which has about 1g of salt).

SWAP ▶ Chocolate muffin

Per shop-sized serving: calories 495; fat 26.3g; sugars 35.3g; salt 0.6g

A chocolate muffin is among the best examples of how a single breakfast snack can bump up your daily fat, sugar and calorie intake without you realising it. Munch one of these every morning and you will consume one-quarter of your daily calories if you are a woman (one-fifth if you are a man) and more than one-third of your daily sugars. Plus, the product is 21.9 per cent fat and is therefore deemed a high-fat food, so it is clearly one to overlook in the pastry cabinet.

FOR ▶ Pain au chocolat

Per shop-sized serving: calories 270; fat 15.1g; sugars 7.1g; salt 0.7g

If it's chocolate you're after, this is a far better option than a chocolate muffin. Although the pastry means its fat content is 23 per cent, you save considerably on the calories and sugar (11 per cent of the weight compared with 29.4 per cent sugars in the muffin) while still getting that chocolate fix.

SWAP ▶ Almond croissant

Per shop-sized serving: calories 350; fat 19.8g; sugars 11.3g; salt 0.5g

A butter croissant filled with a sweet almond paste and coated with icing sugar and flaked almonds, puts this croissant in a high band for its 23.9 per cent fat content, most of which (16.2 per cent) is saturated fat. Of the most popular types of croissants, only pain au raisin contains more calories.

FOR ▶ Apricot croissant

Per shop-sized serving: calories 260; fat 11.3g; sugars 8.0g; salt 0.5g

Although the apricot doesn't make this sugar-glazed pastry with sweet crème pâtissière a healthy option, the overall profile of the pastry is an improvement on the almond one. Indeed, it contains almost half the fat of an almond croissant and less sugar, while saving 90 calories to boot. Reserved for an occasional treat, it is a better choice.

————

SWAP ▸ Cheese twist pastry

Per shop-sized serving: calories 316; fat 18.3g; sugars 3.8g; salt 0.5g

Being savoury, this Cheddar and Emmenthal-filled pastry might seem a better option, but it's 24.1 per cent fat – very high.

FOR ▸ Wholemeal muffin

Per shop-sized serving: calories 130; fat 1.4g; sugars 2.3g; salt 0.5g

This muffin is reasonably filling and yet among the lowest in both fat and calories. Wholemeal muffins have a denser texture than those made with white flour but provide a fibre boost. Top with cottage cheese or another low-fat cream cheese to add moisture and flavour without packing on the fat. Compared to the cheese twist, you get 186 fewer calories and 16.9g less fat before a topping is added.

Breakfast sandwiches

Hot sandwiches, muffins and panini are among the most popular takeaway breakfast choices from cafés, coffee shops and fast-food outlets. Certainly, they can smell tempting as you queue to buy your morning coffee. But be warned that some ready-made and hot sandwiches contain as much salt as nine bags of crisps and are also high in fat and calories. Even at breakfast time, you'll find panini contain dressings and sauces laden with oil and mayonnaise, and this is often the reason why a sandwich can be transformed into an unhealthy feast. With 110 calories and 12g of fat per tablespoon, 80 per cent of mayonnaise is fat – and it crops up with alarming regularity in pre-prepared breakfasts. Often home-made versions can be far healthier options. Grilled bacon between slices of freshly sliced bread served alongside a couple of grilled tomatoes comprises a considerably lower fat and salt breakfast compared with the commercially assembled variety. But if you are tempted to grab a sandwich on the run, take care when choosing, because many of those typically on offer at well-known chains are not everything they seem.

SWAP ▶ All-day breakfast club sandwich

Per shop-sized serving: calories 592; fat 20.9g; sugars 9.7g; salt 4.25g

This hot sandwich has the most calories of all the breakfast meals tested and more than a quarter of daily energy needs. It is also very high in salt, providing almost 75 per cent of the GDA, and contains almost one-third of your daily saturated fat intake. It's not all bad news – it has less overall fat than a blueberry muffin and less saturated fat than a pain au raisin – but this should be a very occasional treat. You'd be much better off with a grilled bacon sandwich on unbuttered wholemeal bread.

FOR ▶ Egg, bacon and mushroom breakfast panini

Per shop-sized serving: calories 269; fat 9.0g; sugars 3.6g; salt 3g

Ciabatta bread stuffed with an egg, mayonnaise, roasted mushrooms, bacon and tomato ketchup looks as if it should be more calorific. In fact, it contains less than half the calories in a typical all-day breakfast club sandwich and is not particularly high in fat. The bacon and bread together contain half the recommended daily salt intake, but the mushrooms add to the fibre count and the egg provides some iron and vitamins A, D and E.

SWAP ▸ Bacon, lettuce and tomato sandwich (BLT)

Per shop-sized serving: calories 471; fat 27.2g; sugars 5.5g; salt 2g

The lettuce and tomato do little to redeem this sandwich, which is shockingly high in salt and fat, and provides nearly a quarter of a woman's daily calories. Bacon, butter and mayonnaise bump up the fat content.

FOR ▸ Bacon and ketchup breakfast muffin

Per shop-sized serving: calories 277; fat 7.5g; sugars 2.2g; salt 2.5g

Of the coffee shop options, a bacon muffin is among the better choices. Its relatively low fat and calorie content are partly due to its smaller size than many of the paninis and toasted sandwiches. Not great on the salt front, but a reasonable option and it saves 194 calories compared to the BLT.

SWAP ▸ Ham and cheese croissant

Per shop-sized serving: calories 378; fat 21g; sugars 4.8g; salt 1.5g

Add ham and cheese to a buttery croissant and you are never going to be looking at a low-fat breakfast. This contains considerably more fat than a bacon butty.

FOR ▶ Ham and egg muffin

Per shop-sized serving: calories 314; fat 12.2g; sugars 0.9g; salt 1.5g

Although not a low-fat choice, a ham and egg muffin does contain almost half the amount of the ham and cheese croissant and considerably less sugar. Choose a wholemeal muffin where available and you will bump up the fibre content slightly.

DID YOU KNOW?

Scientists from the University of Newcastle have showed that bacon sandwiches can help to cure a hangover by speeding up the metabolism and helping the body to get rid of the alcohol more quickly. (Using wholemeal bread is the best option.)

Hot breakfast favourites

Despite an influx of newcomers on the takeaway breakfast front, traditional meals remain as popular as ever both on eat-in menus and as weekend or occasional treats at home. Many hail from an era when substantial calorie intakes were required to fuel energy expenditure and should really be reserved for occasional treats in these days of minimal physical movement. Still, many options are not as loaded with fat and salt as their trendier rivals and can form a surprisingly balanced and nutrient-packed meal at any time of the day.

SWAP ▶ Grilled smoked kipper

Per 145g (5oz) serving: calories 215; fat 16.5g; salt 1.8g

Kippers are whole herrings that have been split from tail to head and gutted, then smoked. Herrings and kippers are a good source of omega-3 fats shown to have a host of health benefits including helping to prevent heart disease. Beware though – smoked kippers are very high in fat and salt, so limit how often you have them to once a week at the most. Oily fish such as kippers are generally a good choice, but it is always better to opt for non-smoked fish whenever possible. You will make calorie savings if you swap them though.

FOR ▶ Scrambled egg (made with 2 eggs) with smoked salmon

Calories 185; fat 12g; sugars 0.1g; salt 1.75g

As well as other nutrients, eggs yolks contain lutein and zeax-anthin, which could help to prevent or even reverse the age-related eye problem macular degeneration (MD). This is one of the leading causes of blindness and occurs as a consequence of getting older, and a low intake of lutein is implicated as a risk factor. Salmon is a great source of omega-3 fats – healthy fats that protect the body against heart disease. Serve with some unbuttered, wholemeal toast and cook the eggs without added fat for a wholesome meal. Plus, you save 70 calories by making this swap.

––––––––

SWAP ▶ Full English fry-up

Calories 618; fat 37g; sugar 21g; salt 3.5g

The nutritional calculation above is based on one fried egg, one rasher of bacon, one sausage, a spoonful of baked beans, half a grilled tomato and a piece of fried bread but start doubling up on some of these – as many people do – and you could easily exceed your daily recommended fat intake. Grilling instead of frying the bacon and sausage will reduce the total fat, as will poaching the egg rather than frying it. Better still, swap it altogether.

FOR ▶ 2 poached eggs on toast with grilled tomato

Calories 249; fat 12g; sugars 3.1g; salt 1.3g

Eggs contain a wide range of vitamins and minerals, including vitamin D, which promotes mineral absorption and good bone health; iodine, for making thyroid hormones; and phosphorus, which is essential for healthy bones and teeth. Tomatoes are rich in lycopene, a substance that has been shown to protect against some forms of cancer. Poaching is a healthy way of cooking eggs because no extra calories are added. Make these changes, and this swap from a fry-up cuts out a whopping 369 calories – almost a meal in itself.

––––––––––

SWAP ▶ Kedgeree

Per 400g (14oz) serving: calories 673; fat 36g; sugar 12g; salt 3.06g

Many people would think the great British breakfast favourite, kedgeree, is a nutritionally balanced choice, but as it is traditionally made from rice, flaked smoked fish, boiled eggs, parsley, lemon juice, butter and cream it has a tendency to be loaded with fat and calories. It also has more than half the recommended daily intake of salt for an adult; however, the basic ingredients – rice, fish and eggs – are relatively low in fat and highly nutritious. Using low-fat crème fraîche instead of cream, and less or no butter, can reduce the fat content considerably making it a healthier option but you can still improve on the 'full-throttle' version.

FOR ▶ Boiled egg and bread or toast 'soldiers'

Calories 185; fat 5g; sugars trace; salt trace

One egg provides 13 essential nutrients, all in the yolk (egg whites contain albumen, an important source of protein, and no fat). This swap saves 488 calories. Recent studies have shown that eating eggs for breakfast helps to offset hunger pangs more effectively than a high carbohydrate-based cereal. Make your soldiers from wholemeal bread to boost your fibre intake and energy levels. Spread a little butter on the soldiers.

THE TOP 5 BREAKFAST JUICES

One way to boost the nutrient content of your breakfast is to swill down your meal with a glass of freshly squeezed fruit juice. Fruit and vegetable juices have long been known to boost immunity and help to fight off colds and viruses. The vitamin C they contain also helps the body to absorb iron from food that is consumed at the same time. As they are high in sugar and are acidic (not good news for the teeth), juices should ideally be limited to one a day. Here is a guide to five of the best health-boosting juices (for more detailed information about juices and their nutritional content, see Chapter 12). From the list below, vary the fruit juices you drink for maximum health effects:

▶

Orange An antioxidant in orange juice, called hesperidin, improves blood vessel function and helps lower a person's risk of heart disease. Men who drank 500ml (18fl oz) of orange juice (containing 292mg of hesperidin) daily had improved heart health and lower blood pressure than those who drank a hesperidin-fortified drink, suggesting that orange juice might contain other benefits as well as the hesperidin. It is also known that supplements of citrate, a substance found in citrus juices, can help to slow the formation of kidney stones, but some people find the acidic nature of these supplements hard to tolerate and the natural food is better. A daily glass of orange juice produces similar benefits.

Apple Drinking apple juice may help to prevent the decline of an essential neurotransmitter called acetylcholine, the presence of which is critical for memory and brain health. Although the study was conducted on mice, the researchers claimed that an intake of two glasses – 500ml (18fl oz) in total – of apple juice a day could have similar benefits in adults. Apple juice also aids digestion and healthy bowel movements.

Tomato Lycopene, the substance that makes tomatoes red, is effective at mopping up particles called free radicals, which can damage the body's tissues. A regular consumption of tomatoes, particularly in processed, juiced or cooked form, which enhances absorption by the body, is linked to a reduction in prostate cancer. Evidence is inconclusive but promising enough for many cancer experts

▶

to encourage men to increase the amount of tomatoes in their diet.

Pineapple The enzyme bromelain, found in the pineapple plant and juice of the fruit, is said to help the body to digest proteins. When taken on an empty stomach, bromelain is understood to act as an anti-inflammatory agent, which may reduce arthritis joint pain and swelling. A combination of enzymes that include bromelain may be a safe alternative to anti-inflammatory drugs for people with mild knee osteoarthritis.

Carrot A compound in carrots, called falcarinol, could have many health benefits. Falcarinol is a natural pesticide found in carrots that protects carrots from fungal diseases; in the human diet, carrots are its only source. Animal studies have shown that falcarinol results in a one-third lower risk of developing colorectal cancer.

CHAPTER **SIX**

■

Coffee break

TWENTY YEARS AGO YOU WOULD have been hard-pushed to find a specialist coffee shop. Now, they are so engrained in our culture that we have become a generation of coffee connoisseurs. Most of us know the difference between a latte and a cappuccino, a flat white and an Americano. What is less well known, however, is the extent to which our coffee break habit is triggering waistbands to expand.

The consumption of liquid calories has increased in parallel with the rise in obesity. Non-alcoholic beverages, of which coffee is a main player, are now estimated to account for almost one-quarter of the calorie intake and to supply half the added sugar consumed by people in the West. Anyone who thinks they should feel dietary virtue for stopping off at a branch of Starbucks, Costa or any other coffee chain rather than McDonald's or Pizza Hut is wrong. Indeed, the fat, calories and sugar we now consume in liquid form are becoming as big a culprit as between-meal snacks when it comes to their potential to lead to weight gain.

You wouldn't consider indulging in a quarter-pounder

between breakfast and lunch, yet it's perfectly possible to get in excess of 500 calories in a hot or iced coffee-shop drink. Some contain no coffee at all and are little more than cream, artificial flavourings and lots of sugar and sweetening ingredients. Psychologically, people fail to make an adjustment for liquid calories in the same way they do for extra calories consumed in food. Studies have proven this: when people have been given an additional 450 daily calories in the form of jelly beans, they cut down on other food they would normally consume to avoid weight gain. When they were given a 450-calorie drink, they didn't make the same changes and so consumed far more energy than they normally would in a typical day.

All in all, it's hardly surprising that women who visit coffee shops two to seven times a week have been shown to consume an average 206 calories and 32g of sugar a day more than their non-coffee-drinking counterparts. Over time, their cuppa habit would almost certainly have an adverse effect on their weight. Considering that a plain cup of coffee contains only two calories (and no fat), there are ways to avoid the hefty gains that come when it is dressed up with unnecessary extras. This guide will help you select safely.

Hot drinks

Whether your preference is for skinny or whipped, with an extra shot of caffeine or a pump of syrup, the likelihood is that your favourite beverage secretly harbours more calories, fat and sugar than you might imagine. Whereas plain, instant coffee or tea made with a bag was once the favourite daily cuppa, we have developed a growing love affair with gourmet beverages such as lattes, cappuccinos and spiced teas. All of these can be surprisingly bad news for our weight and health. Even drinks made at home can be sugary disasters. Look out for sweetened herbal teas and avoid adding extra teaspoons of sugar, honey or syrups to your home-made drinks. Canned tea and coffee, another coffee genre with rising popularity, are also likely to be full of sugar and little else.

DID YOU KNOW?

A reduction of one daily sweetened and milky coffee-shop drink was associated with a weight loss of 500g (1lb 2oz) at 6 months and 680g (1½lb) at 18 months in one study where participants kept food diaries.

SWAP ▶ Cappuccino (medium with whole milk)

Per serving: calories 140; fat 7g; sugars 9.4g; salt 0.22g

A mix of steamed and foamed milk added to an espresso shot. If you don't want to swap, ask for a 'skinny' cappuccino made with skimmed milk, which will remove the fat and cut the calories to 82 in a large drink. Sprinkle on cinnamon instead of chocolate powder to save a further 6 calories. Better still, swap it.

FOR ▶ Flat white (medium with whole milk)

Per serving: calories 118; fat 5.8g; sugars 8.1g; salt trace

A relative newcomer on the block in coffee shops, the flat white originates from Australia and is a small, strong white coffee, made with two to three shots of espresso topped with very creamy, well-frothed milk. Unlike lattes and milk coffee drinks, which are served in anything up to a 600ml (20fl oz/1 pint) cup by coffee chains, the flat white is usually served in a 150ml (5fl oz/¼ pint) or 175ml (6fl oz) cup. The milk needs to be very well stretched and spun to make sure it has plenty of tight bubbles – a micro foam – which makes it taste creamy but without the addition of cream itself. It saves you 22 calories and 2.8g of fat when you have it in place of a cappuccino.

———

SWAP ▸ Medium caramel macchiato (medium with skimmed milk)

Per serving: calories 139; fat 1g; sugars 30.6g; salt 0.32g

Caramel and other flavoured macchiatos are a different drink altogether from the simple macchiato and are sweetened and topped with syrups and caramel. Opt for a large one made with whole milk and you are looking at 352 calories and 14.6g of fat. All varieties have about 30g of total sugars per medium mug.

FOR ▸ Double macchiato (with skimmed milk)

Per serving: calories 13; fat trace; sugars 0.3g; salt trace

Made from an espresso shot topped with foamed milk, the calories are not much higher than a straight espresso. Even with whole milk, the fat content is negligible and the calories 15 per serving. Swap the caramel version for this one and you'll cut 125 calories per cup.

TOP SWAP TIP

- Ask for skimmed, non-fat milk (known as a 'skinny' in coffee-shop lingo). By sticking to skimmed milk, you can cut the calories in your large latte to 160 (122 in a

▶

small size), reduce saturated fat to zero and still provide a healthy dose (450mg) of calcium.

- Skip the whip: in many coffee shops, whipped cream adds 80–120 calories and 7g of bad fat that you could do without.

- Remember that sugar (10 calories per sachet) and syrups (70 calories per shot) bump up your total. Some coffee shops have sugar-free syrups made with artificial sweeteners, so if you must have sweetness ask for those.

- Low-fat, milky drinks are a good choice, as they contribute about 200mg of calcium to the recommended daily total of 800–1,000mg. Among the best sources are skimmed milk latte (320mg of calcium), and skimmed café mocha (277mg of calcium)

- Avoid sugary toppings: chocolate and caramel on top of your drink add 6–15 calories.

- If it's a caffeine kick you're after, opt for a single shot espresso. Even if you add sugar (10 calories per sachet), this pure coffee shot and water offers the lowest calorie coffee option on the menu.

SWAP ▶ Latte (medium with whole milk)

Per serving: calories 223; fat 11.5; sugars trace

The latte is a surprisingly poor choice. A large latte – made from 1–2 shots of espresso with steamed milk – contains almost one-quarter the daily recommended fat intake for women and much of it is of the saturated variety. If you are not careful, your drink could balloon to a whole-milk vanilla latte containing 380 calories and 14.5g of fat in each large cup.

FOR ▶ Americano (medium)

Per serving: calories 8; fat none; sugars none; salt none

Made from 2–3 espresso shots topped with water. Most people add milk to their Americano – and that's no bad thing. Whereas a few studies have suggested that a high intake of caffeine promotes the leeching of calcium from bones, adding milk to your cuppa will offset any such risk (see Caffeine – Good or Bad?). Swap to this and you save 215 calories and 11.5g of fat.

CAFFEINE – GOOD OR BAD?

Whether or not caffeine is good for us is a hotly debated topic among scientists. Caffeine acts as a stimulant to the heart and central nervous system and is also known to increase blood pressure in the short term, although there's no conclusive evidence of long-term effects on blood pressure. Women should consume less than 200mg of caffeine a day during pregnancy according to the UK Department of Health, this represents about two cups of instant coffee or tea; however, it is generally accepted that, unless otherwise advised by your doctor, it is safe to consume the equivalent of four to six cups of instant or moderately strong coffee a day. Morning coffee, in particular, can enhance alertness. Drinking four cups over the course of a morning has been shown to help people to work more efficiently. A study published in the *Journal of the American Medical*

▶

Association reported that men who drink two to three cups of coffee a day had a 40 per cent lower risk of developing gallstones than non-coffee drinkers.

If you already lead a stressful lifestyle, though, your coffee habit could make things worse. At Duke University in the US it was discovered that people who drink four cups in the morning had slightly elevated blood pressure levels and greater amounts of stress hormones during the day. And several studies have shown that the consumption of five or more cups a day is a risk factor for osteoporosis, because a heavy caffeine intake may interfere with calcium absorption. On the other hand, the same findings have often proved that the negative effects of calcium loss can be offset by adding a tablespoon of milk to your cuppa. The National Osteoporosis Society says there is no conclusive evidence that coffee thins bones, but advises no more than five cups to be safe. Those trying to break the caffeine habit can find that withdrawal symptoms can occur after regular consumption of just two-and-a-half to three cups a day. Caffeinism, as it is sometimes called, manifests as headaches, migraine and sickness. Here's where you can expect to find caffeine:

- Mug of instant coffee: 100mg

- Mug of filter coffee: 140mg

- Mug of tea: 75mg

- Can of cola: 40mg

- Can of energy drink: 80mg

- Small 50g (1¾oz) bar of plain (dark) chocolate: about 50mg

- Small 50g (1¾oz) bar of milk chocolate: about 25mg

SWAP ▶ White chocolate mocha (medium with whole milk)

Per serving: calories 500; fat 18.7g; sugars 58.6g; salt trace

A large white chocolate mocha with whipped cream is more of a dessert than a drink. It is made from espresso (although you can barely detect the coffee taste) and white chocolate sauce topped with steamed milk and sweetened whipped cream. In calorie and fat terms you would be better off gobbling a burger with cheese. And it has more than half the total daily maximum of sugars for a woman.

FOR ▶ Mocha (medium with skimmed milk)

Per serving: calories 132; fat 1g; sugars 23.4g; salt trace

Made with three-quarters steamed milk, a pump of chocolate sauce and two shots of espresso, this is a preferable way to get your sugar shot compared with many of the highly sweetened beverages on offer. Add whipped cream, though, and you are looking at over 300 calories per cup.

SWAP ▶ Hot chocolate with whipped cream (medium with whole milk)

Per serving: calories 549; fat 27g; sugars 47g; salt trace

A large hot chocolate with cream has the calories and fat content of three hot dogs. It also provides more than half a woman's daily sugar intake and nearly one-third of a man's. Even worse is a white hot chocolate, which contains a whopping 719 calories and 33.4g of fat in a large mug. That is more than you would get in a burger chain coffee served with 12 of their creamers and 32 packets of sugar.

FOR ▶ Hot chocolate (medium with skimmed milk, no cream)

Per serving: calories 217; fat 1.9g; sugars 40.1g; salt trace

Reduce the serving size, switch to skimmed milk and cut out the cream, and you can sip a hot chocolate in the knowledge that it contains 13 times less fat. It is still a highly sweetened drink, but less of an indulgence than the whipped cream variety. Save 332 calories.

DID YOU KNOW?

Be aware that some chains, instead of using milk, make drinks such as hot chocolate with a mix that is largely sugar and non-dairy creamer (containing the extremely unhealthy partially hydrogenated soybean oil and yet more sugar). Often, they don't make this clear and it's worth asking how the drink is made and with which ingredients, if you are a regular. Some chains have detailed information about ingredients and sources on websites – a useful resource.

SWAP ▶ Chai tea latte (medium with whole milk)

Per serving: calories 193; fat 5.0g; sugars 31.3g; salt none

Tea has a healthy reputation because of its antioxidant content, but any nutrient benefits are offset by fat and sugar in this drink. In a large version of the drink, which is sweetened with honey, there are as many calories as a cheese sandwich. If you want to have this drink, choose a milk-free iced tea (black or green) which will supply just 80 calories and no saturated fat. Or swap it.

FOR ▶ Breakfast tea (medium with whole milk and sugar)

Per serving: calories 15; fat 0.2g; sugars none; salt none

Black tea contains some useful minerals such as zinc, manganese and potassium, and scientists are researching its potential to reduce the risk of coronary heart disease and some cancers. A review of 17 studies concluded that the risk of heart attacks was 11 per cent lower, on average, when people drank three cups of bog-standard black tea each day. It has also been shown to lower blood pressure when consumed regularly. Swap to this and save 178 calories and 31g of sugars.

TOP SWAP TIP

It would seem that switching to green tea is an excellent choice to make, as shown by more than two decades worth of evidence backing its health benefits (although most of it, admittedly, was conducted in test tubes, not on humans). Although not caffeine-free, green tea has half the caffeine content of black tea. Among the most well-reported benefits is the tea's rich flavonoid content – powerful antioxidants found in high concentrations in both green and black teas. The concentration of the compounds depends on how long the tea has been brewed. It has been suggested that drinking at least two cups of green

▶

tea daily inhibits cancer growth. Of the few human studies that have been done, one showed that increased green tea consumption before and after surgery was associated with lower recurrence of stage-1 and stage-2 breast cancer in 500 women.

Researchers also think it's good for the heart. Drinking at least four cups of green tea every day was shown to reduce the severity of coronary heart disease among men in one trial, while another study of more than 3,000 men and women found that the more of the tea consumed the less severe the clogging of the heart's blood vessels. It can even help to cure bad breath – the polyphenols it contains destroy a number of compounds in the mouth that can lead to bad breath.

Iced drinks

Chilled and iced drinks have become a staple on the menus of coffee shops. Some are merely cold versions of traditional coffees, but more often than not they contain no coffee at all and are more like glorified milk shakes than anything else. As with the hot versions of these drinks, look out for sweet syrups, sweetened creams and added sugar. Indeed, the World Cancer Research Fund has warned that some iced coffees contain so many calories and so much fat that they increase people's chances of becoming overweight, the second biggest cause of cancer. Watch out that you are not consuming the calorific equivalent of a main meal in each refreshing drink you grab to go. If your drink has over 400 calories, that equates to about 20 per cent of a typical woman's daily calorie needs.

SWAP ▶ Vanilla iced coffee (medium with whole milk)

Per serving: calories 340; fat 15.6g; sugars 44.7g; salt trace

A blended crème drink made from a coffee-free mix of sugar, syrup, milk and ice topped with whipped cream. Blended crème drinks are a variation on the original iced coffee which is made from a mix of coffee, sugar, milk and ice. The addition of syrups and flavourings, however, turn the drink into a dieter's disaster. If you want to have an iced coffee, skip the whipped cream and you will save 131 calories for a large one. Choose a small, low-fat iced coffee with no cream, and your calories amount to only 119. Better still, swap it.

FOR ▶ Iced vanilla latte (medium with whole milk)

Per serving: calories 255; fat 3.9g; sugars 36.6g; salt trace

An espresso-based drink that is blended with vanilla syrup and 'diluted' with ice. If it's a vanilla chill you are after, this is a far better choice than the vanilla iced coffee, containing less than one-quarter of the fat per serving. Save 85 calories with this swap.

SWAP ▶ Strawberry-and-cream iced drink with whipped cream (medium with whole milk)

Per serving: calories 415; fat 15.1g; sugars 65.4g; salt trace

Don't be fooled by the mention of fruit in the title – such drinks have rarely been introduced to a whole strawberry. Rather, they are made with a strawberry-flavoured sweet syrup blended with milk, ice and topped with sweetened cream. As a result this contains two-thirds of the daily total sugar intake for a woman.

FOR ▶ Strawberry blended milkshake (medium with whole milk)

Per serving: calories 316; fat 4.8g; sugars 43.8g; salt trace

Although made with similar ingredients and no fresh fruit, a coffee shop 'frappe' milkshake provides considerable savings on fat and some on sugars. This swap saves nearly 100 calories and, although it still contains a lot of sugar, the drink has considerably less than the strawberry and cream concoction.

SWAP ▶ Iced mocha with whipped cream (medium with whole milk)

Per serving: calories 332; fat 18.9g; sugars 24.2g; salt trace

An espresso shot combined with sweetened mocha (chocolate) sauce on ice and topped with sweetened cream. If you want to have this, cut the cream and you will obviously save some calories and fat. A swap is preferable.

FOR ▶ Iced Americano (medium)

Per serving: calories 17; fat 0g; sugars 0g; salt trace

This is a basic iced coffee to which milk can be added. If it's a caffeine shot with a chill you are after, then this is a good choice. Save over 300 calories with the swap and lose almost 19g of fat and 24g of sugar (unless you add milk, but it will still be considerably less than the iced mocha).

SWAP ▶ Chocolate frappe milkshake (medium with whole milk)

Per serving: calories 317; fat 4.6g; sugars 55g; salt trace

A coffee shop milkshake, containing a rich chocolate sauce, chocolate powder, milk and ice, is not too bad a choice. But there is scope for improvement, especially as it contains 12.1 per cent sugars.

FOR ▶ Latte frappe (medium with whole milk)

Per serving: calories 274; fat 3.9g; sugars 48.7g; salt trace

With 11.4 per cent sugars and 0.9 per cent fat, this is a better choice – although by no means perfect – if you prefer a chilled drink. It is made with an espresso shot, milk and crushed ice. And it saves you 43 calories.

MAKE YOUR OWN

Iced coffee beverages aren't difficult to make: combine coffee, ice, skimmed milk, cocoa powder or cinnamon, and a little sugar. Or whip up a fruit booster with freshly blended fruit (berries are ideal), fruit juice and ice.

SWAP ▶ Caramel iced coffee with whipped cream (medium with whole milk)

Per serving: calories 351; fat 16g; sugars 46.1g; salt trace

One of the worst offenders in the iced drinks ranges, this has over half a woman's recommended daily sugar intake and almost one-quarter of her daily calories. It does contain coffee in the form of an espresso shot, but the sweetness of the caramel sauce mixed with the ice, the sweetened whipped cream and the caramel topping drown out the taste. A sugary horror.

FOR ▸ Espresso iced coffee (medium with whole milk)

Per serving: calories 217; fat 2.1g; sugars 43.8g; salt trace

Not exactly low in sugar, but it does contain slightly less of the sweet stuff and one-seventh of the fat of the caramel drink. You also save calories – just don't drink this one too often.

———————

SWAP ▸ Iced tea latte (medium with whole milk)

Per serving: calories 259; fat 6.9g; sugars 4.2g; salt trace

This sweetened tea drink is positioned towards the healthier end of the chilled drinks' spectrum and is not too bad an option, although you could save on fat by switching to semi- or skimmed milk.

FOR ▸ Mango and passionfruit iced crush (medium)

Per serving: calories 191; fat 0.8g; sugars 45g; salt trace

This gets a gold star for being the healthiest of iced drinks. It is made with 100 per cent fruit juices (although not freshly squeezed – they are from purées) mixed with banana purée. It has no added sugar or sweeteners and the sugars it contains are derived from the fruit juices. Even so, its sugariness means you shouldn't drink it every day. Swap to this, though, and you immediately lose over 6g of fat and 68 calories.

———————

CHECK YOUR SIZES

As with many food chains, coffee shops are guilty of providing huge portion sizes. Some chains now offer 916ml (32fl oz) drinks that dwarf the previous largest measure on offer: 591ml (21fl oz). A 916ml (32fl oz) lemon iced tea provides a colossal 59g of sugar. And the bigger the drink, the higher the calorie, fat and sugar content. If in doubt, opt for a regular serving size.

Coffee shop snacks

Nothing looks quite as alluring as the display of tempting cakes and biscuits to be served alongside your coffee, as you queue for your drink. Coffee chains have become adept at making sure you stand in front of temptation just long enough to start salivating. Pushy baristas are trained to encourage you to indulge. And does it really matter if you do? Many look wholesome – they are made with oats, dried fruit and organic ingredients. Others appear to be small in size and, one might think, would nibble away at only a little of your daily fat and calorie intake; however, coffee shop treats are not what they seem. Served with a milky drink, they can be more calorific and fat-laden than a full English breakfast.

SWAP ▶ Shortbread

Per 2-bar serving: calories 245; fat 14.5g; sugars 8.8g; salt 0.2g

Two bars of coffee shop shortbread comprise almost one-third of their weight in butter and other fats. Sugar levels are acceptable, but there are better snack options, particularly if you are looking for something to eat with a calorific coffee.

FOR ▶ Almond biscotti

Per biscuit: calories 147; fat 5.8g; sugars 8.6g; salt 0.2g

Designed for dunking into your coffee, these hard-baked Italian biscuits, with ground and flaked almonds, are a perfect way to enjoy a long-lasting snack (they take some crunching) and save on calories and fat in the process. Save 98 calories and 8.7g of fat.

———————

SWAP ▶ Granola bar

Per bar: calories 397; fat 22g; sugars 25.4g; salt 0.1g

Don't be fooled into thinking an oat-based granola bar packed with dried fruit and coconut is a healthy option. It might be full of dried apricots, raisins and mixed seeds, but more sugar is added. This is a high fat and sugar snack.

FOR ▶ Palmine biscuit

Per biscuit: calories 75; fat 4.5g; sugars 2.5g; salt 0.1g

These palm-shaped biscuits are newcomers to the coffee-shop shelf. They have a sweet, buttery taste but are relatively low in calories, fat and sugar – a good way to indulge that sweet tooth without too many adverse consequences. The swap saves you 322 calories.

SWAP ▸ Carrot cake

Per shop-sized serving: calories 560; fat 35.4g; sugars 44.1g; salt 0.2g

A classic example of how a healthy-sounding treat is not always the best option. In this case, a slice of carrot cake, topped with buttery icing, provides more than one-quarter of a woman's daily calories (and more than one-fifth of a man's), it has whopping levels of fat and is among the highest in sugar content of all the coffee-shop snacks on sale.

FOR ▸ Rocky road

Per shop-sized serving: calories 420; fat 27g; sugars 27g; salt 0.2g

It may contain marshmallow, biscuit pieces, raisins and chocolate, but you save 140 calories and 8g of fat by opting for this over the carrot cake.

———————

SWAP ▸ Caramel shortcake

Per biscuit: calories 352; fat 19.5g; sugars 29.3g; salt 0.3g

A snack with a sweet and buttery shortcake base, sweet caramel sauce and chocolate is never going to be a low-sugar option. And the fat here is high too.

FOR ▸ Marshmallow chocolate twizzle

Per biscuit: calories 183; fat 6.4g; sugars 27.6g; salt 0g

Marshmallow is a low-fat treat, which means the fat levels in this snack are also low. You don't save much on sugars, partly because it is dipped in sugar strands and chocolate, but it's preferable to many sweet snacks on offer and it spares 169 calories compared to the caramel shortcake.

––––––––––

SWAP ▸ Chocolate flapjack

Per cake: calories 392; fat 18g; sugars 26.1g; salt 0.3g

Despite the benefits of oats – shown to lower cholesterol and boost heart health when eaten regularly – the butter, sugar and syrup in flapjacks load on the fat and calories. In one bar, almost half the fat is saturated and more than a quarter of its weight is sugar. There is less fat in a cheese toastie than in coffee-shop flapjack.

FOR ▸ Oat and raisin cookie

Per biscuit: calories 282; fat 14g; sugars 22.9g; salt 0.2g

If you like the oat taste and texture of a flapjack, this is a better option and it's over 100 calories lighter. The dried fruit it contains contributes to some of the total sugars but also adds a little fibre.

––––––––––

SWAP ▸ Chocolate cheesecake

Per shop-sized serving: calories 533; fat 36g; sugars 38g; salt 0.6g

This has to be among the most calorific of all coffee-shop cakes and pastries. Containing more calories than a decent sandwich, its biscuit base and creamy topping mean it clocks in with 36 per cent fat and 38 per cent sugar. It also contains more salt than many other cakes and biscuits.

FOR ▸ Double chocolate brownie

Per shop-sized serving: calories 314; fat 14.7g; sugars 32.7g; salt 0.2g

Many coffee-shop brownies are sugar-loaded and topped with extra chocolate. But, as hard as it is to swallow, they are a far better bet than creamy cheesecake, with a saving of 219 calories and almost two-thirds less fat.

Herbal teas

Makers of herbal and fruit teas have seen sales rise by 10 per cent in recent years as more people seek to reduce caffeine in their diets. Whereas a traditional black tea from India, Ceylon and Kenya contains almost half as much of the stimulant as instant coffee (there's about 40mg of caffeine per mug compared to 100mg in a mug of instant coffee and 140mg in filter coffee) many herbal teas contain none. The World Health Organization recommends a maximum caffeine intake of under 300mg a day.

Moreover, herbal teas are reputed to have wide-ranging health benefits with naturopaths long recommending them for their medicinal qualities. It's claimed they can help with everything from easing a cold and indigestion to fighting infection and nausea, and while the benefits are largely unproven, the anecdotal evidence is plentiful.

When choosing, make the distinction between herbal and fruit-flavoured teas. It is the former – including thyme, peppermint and ginger – that have the reported therapeutic virtues. Fruit-based teas such as rosehip, apple and orange are enjoyed more for their flavour. Check labels to make sure the tea contains authentic herbs and avoid any with artificial flavourings or additives.

Chamomile Herbalists claim that tea made from the small, golden buds of chamomile encourages sleep, soothes a queasy stomach and relieves heartburn. It is said to contain small amounts of tryptophan, an amino acid known for its tranquil-lising effects, which can help to promote sleep. But when the US Department of Agriculture reviewed scientific literature on the bioactivity of chamomile, they found no human clini-cal trials that examined its calming effect; however, they did produce test-tube evidence that chamomile tea has moderate antimicrobial activity and significant anti-platelet-clumping activity, helping to lower the risk of heart disease if drunk regularly.

Elderflower An effective decongestant, elderflower helps to clear the nasal passages of catarrh. It is also a good diaphoretic; meaning it encourages the body to sweat.

Ginger This warming spice is renowned for easing sickness and queasiness, making it great for morning sickness and travel sickness. It is also said to relieve rheumatic aches and pains by stimulating the circulation.

Rosehip A beautiful pink tea, rosehip is said to stimulate the body and mind. Experts in Chinese medicine believe it has puri-fying and cleansing qualities.

Nettle A great tonic when you are feeling run down, nettle tea has a relatively rich mineral content.

Fennel Don't let the distinctive liquorice flavour put you off; fennel helps to relax the intestinal muscles and is particularly good for constipation, colic and flatulence. Because fennel is a diuretic, it is said to help clean the kidneys.

Peppermint A traditional remedy for nausea and vomiting, peppermint is said to stimulate bile production in the gall bladder, breaking down fat in the digestive system and thereby relieving sickness. Many claim it also helps relieve a blocked nose. In test-tube trials by the US Department of Agriculture, peppermint tea was found to have significant antimicrobial and antiviral activities, as well as strong antioxidant and anti-tumour actions.

Raspberry leaf Also known as red raspberry leaf tea, this is a herbal remedy and not the same as raspberry fruit tea. Drinking two to three cups a day during late pregnancy is reputed to make for an easier labour. The tea is thought to tone the muscles of the uterus (womb) to help it work better during labour.

Hibiscus One of the few teas to have scientific backing for its properties. A human clinical trial on hibiscus tea found that it lowered blood pressure in a group of pre-hypertensive and mildly hypertensive adults.

Spearmint Allegedly good for relieving the symptoms of colds, sinus and upper respiratory conditions.

DID YOU KNOW?

Dentists found that the acidic nature of some varieties of fruit tea can damage tooth enamel. Researchers put extracted teeth in a blackcurrant, ginseng and vanilla tea, a traditional tea, and water. After 14 days, the teeth in

➤

the ordinary tea and the water were virtually unchanged, but the fruit tea had dissolved a layer of enamel from the teeth by several micrometres (thousandths of a millimetre). Traditional herbal teas with no fruit content, like chamomile or peppermint, were not a danger to teeth. Those containing fruits such as lemon, raspberry or blackcurrant appeared to present the risk when the equivalent of three cups a day were consumed over several years.

You might get more than you expected in a cheap herbal or fruit tea. Studies have shown that they often contain unlisted extra ingredients such as weeds, ferns or bits of tree. In one study, 21 of 60 herbal tea products contained rogue ingredients not listed on the labels.

Ordinary 'builder's tea' teabags are one of the largest providers of fluoride in our diets – on average, tea provides up to 70 per cent of our total intake of this mineral, which can help in reducing tooth decay.

CHAPTER **SEVEN**

■

Lunch on the run

OFTEN, LUNCH IS THE MEAL to which we pay the least attention, grabbed on the run in the middle of a hectic day. And perhaps more than any other meal, it seems that there is an impressive array of lunchtime options that will suit your palate and your waistline; however, your lunchtime snacks could secretly harbour more calories and fat than the rest of your daily meals put together. Many seemingly nutritious lunchtime meal choices are laden with unhealthy ingredients that could be adding inches to your waistline over time.

Did you know, for example, that some popular pre-packaged sandwiches contain as much salt as nine bags of crisps and are also high in fat and calories? Or that some supermarket salads are no better than many takeaway meals and can contain more fat and calories than a burger and fries? Dressings and sauces laden with oil and mayonnaise are often the reason why sand-wiches and salads are transformed into an unhealthy feast. With 12g of fat per tablespoon, 80 per cent of mayonnaise is fat – and it crops up with regularity in lunchtime selections.

In short, the lunch that looks to contain the least fat can often be loaded with it, and that seemingly innocent salad can provide a significant chunk of your salt intake. So which lunch to choose?

Sandwiches

Tempted as we might be by the range of lunch choices now available, sandwiches remain our favourite choice in the middle of the day, and traditional fillings still top our preference list. Our number-one sandwich ingredient is chicken – about a third of all the sandwiches we buy contain chicken in one form or another, and the chicken salad sandwich has held the number-one spot for many years. Prawn mayonnaise, egg mayonnaise, and cheese and pickle are also longstanding favourites.

Despite a wide array of different breads being available, 58 per cent of all sandwiches are still made with unimaginative white sandwich bread, and fashionable wraps account for just 4 per cent of the market. With basic ingredients, sandwiches make a balanced meal that can be super-healthy. Include some low-fat protein – egg, ham or chicken – and add some salad ingredients, and you have an all-round range of nutrients. By far the best (and cheapest) sandwich is home-made. Put together two slices of wholemeal bread, some sliced roast chicken, light mayonnaise, one tomato, cucumber and salad leaves and you amass 355 calories, 7.6g of fat (and 1.5g of salt – a considerable saving on most you can buy).

Things start to go awry when various other ingredients are added, and pre-prepared sandwiches are a different ball game altogether. Surveys have shown them to be loaded with salt and fat. When the consumer campaigning organisation Which? analysed the salt content of sandwiches from popular sandwich chains they found some that contained 4.7g of salt – 75 per cent of an adult's daily maximum – and some cheese sandwiches had as much as five teaspoons of sugar added. Check the labels and you will often find that chicken, ham and beef sandwiches contain unnecessary ingredients such as cornflour, salt, water or tapioca starch to bulk up the meat they contain.

SWAP ▸ Chicken Caesar and bacon wrap

Per shop-sized serving: calories 617; fat 29.4g; sugars 1.7g; salt 3.0g

A classic example of how a lunch can be wrong on so many levels. Its fat content comes from the Caesar dressing (which contains a lot of oil), Italian cheese and bacon. And the salt content is way too high, providing half an adult's daily intake.

FOR ▸ Chicken salad wrap

Per shop-sized serving: calories 364; fat 8.3g; sugars 10.1g; salt 1.5g

By omitting the dressings, bacon and cheese you have a really good sandwich that cuts calorie content almost in half and provides almost 75 per cent less fat. Wraps are better if you pick a wholegrain or seeded variety, and make sure you check the sauces or dressing they use on the label, as these condiments can bump up the calories. Wraps can be packed with fat and salt, although any wrap with about this amount of calories is not bad. Sugars are high, but they come from the vegetables, which contain natural sugars locked within the plant cells, and this is far healthier than many lunches.

SWAP ▶ Toasted club sandwich

Per shop-sized serving: calories 534; fat 19.1g; sugars 3.7g; salt 2.8g

Laden with bacon, mayonnaise and oily, creamy dressings to accompany the chicken, this horror contains more calories than almost every other combination and as much as a giant sausage roll. A McDonald's Big Mac contains fewer calories (490). It is also loaded with fat and salt. No single meal should contain more than 2g of salt to stay on the healthy side and there is almost half an adult's daily recommended salt intake in one sitting here – mainly from the bacon and bread. The bacon, butter and dressings, particularly, let it down.

FOR ▶ Cream cheese and smoked salmon bagel

Per shop-sized serving: calories 420; fat 13.1g; sugars 5.0g; salt 2.2g

Bagels can be healthy (pick a seeded variety for a little more fibre) if you choose low-fat fillings, even though they are quite calorific for their size. This is because they weigh more and are denser than conventional bread, as the average bagel contains the same carbohydrate as four slices of bread. Salmon is a good source of heart-friendly omega-3s and, by picking extra-light cream cheese, it can save you approximately 70 calories per 30g (1oz) serving which would bring this calorie count down considerably. Other good fillings include chicken and roasted vegetables.

———

TOP SWAP TIP

Choose sandwiches carefully:

- Buying from sandwich bars, where you can choose the fillings and the bread, is a better bet than ready-made sandwiches.

- Select mayo or butter – not both. A lower calorie option is mustard spread on your bread.

- Fill up on salad ingredients (without the dressing).

- Check the salt content – 1.5g per 100g (3½oz) is high.

SWAP ▶ BLT sandwich

Per shop-sized serving: calories 488; fat 29.9g; sugars 5.2g; salt 2.0g

A BLT sounds and looks healthy, but while the lettuce and tomato are great, a lot of fat comes from the bacon and dressings. Making your own can reduce this considerably: cut the fat off the rashers and grill them, don't fry. Be very wary in buying a BLT from a supermarket or sandwich shop; they can be lunchtime shockers and, like this one, also high in salt.

FOR ▶ Cheese toastie

Per shop-sized serving: calories 308; fat 13.4g; sugars 2.4g; salt 1.9g

Add some salad items, such as tomatoes, olives, onion, sweetcorn or grilled vegetables, to boost your antioxidant vitamin count – all important for a healthy immune system – and the good old cheese toastie is among the best meals around. If you make one at home in a toasted sandwich machine, avoid brushing with butter on the outside; use a low-fat olive oil spray to lubricate the machine instead. Select a wholemeal bread for more fibre. In all, it saves you 108 calories and a whopping 16.5g of fat.

———————

SWAP ▶ Tuna melt toastie

Per shop-sized serving: calories 435; fat 16.5g; sugars 3.5g; salt 2.3g

This toasted cheese and tuna sandwich is often served on white bread or a panini and with mayonnaise added to the tuna. The salt content is higher than many bought sandwiches and so are the calories, bumped up by the fat content. There is also very little fibre unless a salad is added.

FOR ▶ Tomato and mozzarella panini

Per shop-sized serving: calories 390; fat 18.5g; sugars 3.2g; salt 1.5g

Panini are often more calorific than they look, because of their fillings, which usually include cheese, fatty meats and pesto. Even vegetable-based panini that contain courgettes, aubergines and mushrooms, which can be delicious, have been doused in oil before cooking or serving. Try to get a wholegrain variety where possible and include a good, filling, protein source such as grilled chicken or salmon, because these are lower in fat and high in protein, which is known to fill you up for longer. This is not a bad choice in terms of overall calories, as it comes in 142 lighter than the toastie, but it does have a lot of fat, so eat as an occasional treat.

SWAP ▸ Cheddar and pickle baguette

Per shop-sized serving: calories 611; fat 28.1g; sugars 3.3g; salt 1.5g

The humble cheese and pickle sandwich is where many chains fall down by providing ultra-large sandwiches drenched in mayonnaise, such as this one. Don't be fooled that additions like roasted tomatoes make it healthier – often they are drenched in oil. A slice of Cheddar served in a couple of slices of sourdough or a rustic roll with pickle can come in well under 400 calories, however. Or make a swap.

FOR ▸ Egg mayo and cress sandwich

Per shop-sized serving: calories 372; fat 15.1g; sugars 4.1g; salt 1.0g

Eggs contain a wide range of vitamins and minerals including: vitamin D, which promotes mineral absorption and good bone health; iodine, for making thyroid hormones, which are important for regulating metabolism and energy levels; and phosphorus, essential for healthy bones and teeth. Some vitamin C is provided by the cress, although watercress would be better, because it would also add to the iron count. Choose wholemeal bread and this is a very balanced meal with almost half the fat and calories of the Cheddar baguette.

––––––––

SWAP ▸ Ham and eggs bloomer

Per shop-sized serving: calories 599; fat 25.7g; sugars 1.8g; salt 3g

This sandwich can start out well with the basic ingredients of a multigrain bread, ham and free-range egg, but the mustard mayo and butter bump up the calories and fat. There are healthier choices.

FOR ▶ Prawn mayonnaise sandwich

Per shop-sized serving: calories 300; fat 10.6g; sugars 1.4g; salt 1.5g

Prawns are low in fat and a good source of vitamin B_{12}, important for healthy cells, as well as minerals such as iodine and zinc, which support the immune system and production of hormones. They are a great addition to a lunchtime meal, although less so when drenched in mayonnaise. Still, this has half the calories and 15g less fat for your lunch. Crayfish and rocket sandwiches are similar in terms of nutritional content.

SHOULD YOU CHOOSE SUSHI?

Sushi is the lunchtime snack of choice for the discerning foodie, with sales of sushi now outselling some all-time favourite sandwiches, such as cheese and pickle. Sales in the UK of sushi have risen by 21 per cent in the last few years, as our tastes soared for this simple Japanese food made from rice steeped in vinegar and topped with a variety of fish, much of which is raw. But is it a worthy choice?

Many of the ingredients in sushi have health benefits. The Japanese use seaweed in large amounts in their diet because of its concentrated mineral content – up to a quarter of Japanese food contains it to boost flavour. In sushi, dried sheets of seaweed are wrapped around rice

▶

and vegetables to form a mini-parcel. Seaweed is rich in iodine, which is vital for a healthy thyroid, and also copper, calcium, iron and magnesium.

Wasabi, the green paste often served with sushi, is the Japanese equivalent of English mustard. Thought to cleanse the palate, it too could have health benefits. Scientists in Japan have discovered compounds called isothiocyanates in the paste that can help to prevent tooth decay. It has also been found to aid cancer prevention and prevent blood clots, if eaten regularly.

Sushi often contains raw fish. On average, each person in Japan consumes about 100g (3½oz) of fish every day in forms such as sushi, tempura and sashimi. The omega-3 fatty acids in fish are linked to heart protection and improved circulation. It is thought to be one reason why Japanese rates of heart disease remain among the lowest in the world despite an increase in recent years due to the influence of Western lifestyles. Scientists in Japan found that, eaten regularly, sushi dishes could even protect smokers against lung cancer.

For all its plus points, however, sushi is not always low in calories. A small individual pack gives you about 364 calories and 3.6g of fat, which is perfect for lunchtime. But the calories can mount up when you consider that a single, large California roll, containing a crabstick and avocado, can contain 400 calories and 2g of salt. Many lunch boxes contain several of these mini rolls, so it's easy to overdo it without realising it.

One thing to avoid is adding too much soy sauce. Made from fermented soya beans, soy sauce is widely used in

►

Japanese cooking; however, it has a very high salt content and should be avoided by anyone with high blood pressure or who has been told to have a low-sodium diet. But the single sachet of soy sauce, which usually accompanies sushi, can give you 1g of your daily salt maximum of 6g.

Classic lunches

Lunchtime trends come and go, but there are always classics that ride the fashion wave successfully. Many are small in size, and so we assume that they are little more than a quick snack grabbed on the run. In reality, though, they can be dietary disasters. Take an individual pork pie: it has more calories and four times the total fat of a Big Mac burger. Who'd have thought it? Swaps below are listed per portion size.

SWAP ▶ Individual chicken pie

Per portion: calories 460; fat 30.0g; sugars 4.4g; salt 0.75g

The combination of the pastry case and cream filling means that this little number contributes to nearly 50 per cent of a woman's recommended maximum intake for saturated fat – not good news. A home-made chicken pie would mean that you could use alternatives for the cream such as a white sauce or crème fraîche. You could also replace the pastry with a mashed potato topping and add vegetables to the pie for extra filling. A vegetable pie offers more vitamins but less protein unless it also contains cheese (as many do), but check that it isn't filled with an equally fat-laden cheese sauce, which would offset the benefits.

FOR ▸ Hummus with vegetable sticks

Per portion: calories 117; fat 3.9g; sugars 4.1g; salt 0.12g

You can't get much better than this. Made from chickpeas, which are a good source of protein and carbohydrate, hummus is a very healthy choice. A low-fat hummus will cut calories and fat (although the standard version is low fat compared to many meals), and if you add a pocket of wholemeal pitta bread to provide some carbohydrates to fill you up, it will still come to about 300 calories less than a chicken pie and a fraction of the fat.

———————

SWAP ▸ Cornish pasty

Per portion: calories 467; fat 31.5g; sugars 2.3g; salt 1.2g

Pasties are enjoying something of a resurgence with gourmet pasty shops cropping up everywhere. Pasties should be eaten only as an occasional treat due to their enormously high fat content and calorie values. A typical Cornish pasty contains minced beef and vegetables encased in shortcrust or puff pastry. In traditional pasties, diced steak and chunky vegetables are used, but in commercial varieties the vegetables in a meat pasty are minimal. A vegetable pasty would be better, but they often come with cheese, which bumps up the fat although it does also provide a valuable source of protein.

FOR ▸ Baked potato and chilli

Per portion: calories 460; fat 15.6g; sugars 2.0g; salt 1.6g

Baked potatoes on their own have quite a high GI, or glycaemic index, meaning they offer only a short energy burst; however, the glycaemic load of the meal can be reduced by combining it with a low-GI filling so that it offers a more sustained boost to get you through the afternoon slump. Chilli made with meat and plenty of pulses is an excellent example as long as it is cooked with only a small amount of oil. Using moist fillings like chilli, cottage cheese or baked beans, also means you can avoid adding butter to your baked potato. It contains half the fat of the pasty for a decent plateful.

———————

SWAP ▸ Individual pork pie

Per portion: calories 535; fat 35.1g; sugars 4.2g; salt 1.9g

A whopping one-quarter of the weight of an individual-sized pie is fat included in the fat-laden pastry and processed meat within, and it supplies more than half the recommended daily maximum for a woman's saturated fat intake – 20g (¾oz). With so much fat and carbohydrate in the pastry it is unlikely to fill you up, as fat is known to be less satiating than protein, which means you'll end up eating more at lunch.

FOR ▸ Ploughman's lunch

Per portion: calories 482; fat 25.7g; sugars 2.4g; salt 1.91g

A ploughman's lunch is a good choice *if* you select carefully. Big slabs of cheese and butter would mean calories can soar to levels similar to those provided in a plate of fries. Increase the green salad and tomatoes, and add an apple to make it healthier. Try to select low-fat cheese, such as Edam, or medium-fat cheeses, such as Brie, Camembert, Emmenthal or feta instead of the higher fat cheeses, like Caerphilly, Cheddar, Cheshire, Double Gloucester and Stilton. Even with Cheddar, you have a complete meal for about 50 calories and 10g of fat less than a paltry pork pie.

———————

Soups

Fresh soups with a home-made feel have become a lunchtime favourite in recent years. Sold in the chiller compartment, they seem so much more wholesome than the tinned and dried powder soups, which were the only varieties commercially available for years. In reality, there is not a huge amount of difference between the many branded soups regardless of how they are packaged.

One thing to look out for is their salt content. Although manufacturers have made an effort to cut down on the amount of sodium added to their products in recent years (there has been a reduction of about 17 per cent on average), many are still woefully high. Surveys by the medical lobbying group, Consensus Action on Salt and Health, found that many soups sold in high street chains contain more salt per portion than adults should consume in an entire day (6g). One Thai chicken curry soup had an enormous 8.07g of salt per portion, the same amount as three Big Macs and fries.

Fat contents tend not to be high in soups unless they are made with a lot of cream and cheese. Tomato and vegetable-based broths make the best choices, but a good soup is a nutritious meal all round, provided you select well.

Home-made is simple and best

As always, you are better off making your own soup at home. And it is a true convenience food: chuck in the ingredients, add stock and wait for your steaming bowl of nutrients.

The values of swaps are per 100g (3½oz). Remember, however, that portion sizes vary, and that the actual calorie and fat content could be much higher. Typically, a serving will be 200–300g so take this into account when calculating values. Adding a dollop of cream, cheese or croutons could add 50–100 calories per serving to your soup, so avoid the trimmings.

SWAP ▶ Cream of carrot and coriander

Per 100g (3½oz) serving: calories 54; fat 4.1g; sugar 2.1g; salt 0.6g

Cream of carrot and coriander is not a bad choice. Boiling and puréeing the carrots breaks down the rigid cell structure of the vegetable, which means that maximum levels of beta-carotene, important for a healthy immune system, are released. It's also a good source of vitamin C. This is a healthy choice for fat and sugar, but there's an even lower one.

FOR ▶ Organic three bean soup

Per 100g (3½oz) serving: calories 55; fat 0.9g; sugar 1.1g; salt 0.6g

Beans and pulses are a great soup addition and do wonders for boosting energy levels midday, as they have a low glycaemic index and contain soluble fibre. Beans are also a good source of vitamin B, important for energy production, and the vegetables the soup contains boost vitamin C. Bean-based soups are among the best choices, because they provide filling protein (in the pulses) and fibre and are generally tomato-based so are low in fat. However, both of the soup options contain relatively high levels of salt and – as ever – you'd be better off making your own.

———

SWAP ▶ Bacon and sweetcorn chowder

Per 100g (3½oz) serving: calories 115; fat 8.0g; sugar 1.2g;
salt 0.6g

This type of creamy chowder contains almost 500 calories per
serving and comprises 8.2 per cent fat. A portion would also
provide one-third of an adult's salt intake for a whole day. It
contains sweetcorn, which provides some vitamin C.

FOR ▶ Creamy chicken

Per 100g (3½oz) serving: calories 79; fat 4.8g; sugar 1.4g;
salt 0.5g

Given that this soup is described as 'creamy' you might be
forgiven for thinking this is a poor choice, but in terms of
calories and fat it's not bad, especially soups from Caffé Nero.
Their portion sizes are larger than some chains (there are 316
calories in a serving). And it seems your mother was right:
chicken soup really might help improve the symptoms of a cold
or flu. Researchers in the medical journal *Chest* showed that
chicken soup had anti-inflammatory properties that acted to
stop our throats becoming sore and helped stop the movement
of neutrophils (white blood cells that encourage the flow of
mucus that accumulates in the lungs and nose).

————

SWAP ▶ Broccoli and stilton

Per 100g (3½oz) serving: calories 42; fat 2g; sugar 1.1g;
salt 0.6g

Made with 35–40 per cent broccoli, potatoes, cream and 4–5
per cent Stilton (which raises the fat, although not to high
levels), this is a reasonably wholesome choice, as it provides
plenty of bone-boosting calcium in the cheese and cream. But
you could go one better.

FOR ▶ Mushroom

Per 100g (3½oz) serving: calories 40; fat 1.3g; sugar 0.9g;
salt 0.7g

Mushrooms, a useful source of iron and folate, make up around
25 per cent of this soup, and the other ingredients are onions,
cream, flour and wine. It sounds as if it should contain more
calories, but it is a surprisingly healthy lunchtime choice. Only
its salt content lets it down with one-third of the daily adult
intake per bowlful.

SWAP ▶ Cream of tomato (canned)

Per 100g (3½oz) serving: calories 59; fat 3g; sugar 5g;
salt 0.6g

Tomato soup is a good source of the carotenoid lycopene (and
this one contains 84 per cent of the fruit), which is linked to
lower rates of cancers including breast and prostate. It could
also stem your appetite. Researchers showed that tomato soup
helped people cut down their subsequent calorie intake during
the day. But there is a better choice for lunch.

FOR ▶ Minestrone (canned)

Per 100g (3½oz) serving: calories 33; fat 0.2g; sugar 1.8g; salt 0.6g

Among the lowest in fat and calories of all the soups and yet packed with plenty of filling ingredients. This contains 25 per cent tomatoes, pasta, carrots, onions, celery, swede and peppers. All for fewer calories than even cream of tomato – and virtually no fat.

Salads

Today, ready-to-go salads contain more exotic-sounding ingredients than ever before and are generally considered a way to ensure your lunch is spot-on nutritionally. But many supermarket and coffee-chain salads are so laden with mayonnaise, oily dressings and cheese that they contain more fat and calories than a burger and fries. About 80 per cent of mayonnaise is fat and many salads contain several spoonfuls. Others list oily dressings as constituting almost one-third of the salad's weight.

If you do choose a ready-made salad, try to opt for one that has the dressing served in a separate carton and use it sparingly, if at all. Look out for ingredients like Cheddar cheese and Stilton, cream and other dressings that add to the fat content. Opt instead for a combination of protein – eggs, seafood, lean meat – and unrefined carbohydrates such as brown rice, grains and pasta to fill you up alongside your healthy leaves. Values below are per 100g (3½oz) for the sake of comparison, although remember that portion sizes are generally larger.

SWAP ▶ Caesar salad

Per 100g (3½oz): calories 220; fat 19.0g; sugars 0.2g; salt 0.5g

A traditional Caesar salad uses cos (or Romaine) lettuce that has little nutrient content. Caesar dressing is often laden with fat, and the deep-fried croutons are an additional source of fat. There is protein in the cheese and chicken, if you have it, but a standard portion contains a whopping 45g of fat and, with 19 per cent of its weight from fat, it has a high fat content.

FOR ▶ Salade Niçoise

Per 100g (3½oz): calories 165; fat 8.4g; sugars 1.2g; salt 0.5g

There are a lot of good things in a salade Niçoise, including the boiled egg, green beans and piles of lettuce leaves. Adding peppers, tomatoes and parsley significantly increases the vitamin C content. Fresh tuna (as opposed to canned) has a larger supply of omega-3 fatty acids, which have powerful anti-inflammatory properties. The dressing and olives raise the fat level, but it's still not too high in fat and contains about 413 calories a portion. At home, check the label to make sure a low-fat dressing is not packed with chemicals – if so, stick to a drizzle of olive oil. A salade Niçoise saves you 24g of fat and almost 140 calories over a Caesar.

SWAP ▶ Mozzarella and tomato salad with pesto dressing

Per 100g (3½oz): calories 155; fat 7.9g; sugar 1.5g; salt 0.3g

A pasta-based salad with mozzarella, rocket leaves and a pot of pesto dressing served separately. With 276 calories per portion, it is a reasonable lunchtime choice, although it has more fat than needed.

FOR ▶ Chicken salad with Caesar dressing

Per 100g (3½oz): calories 92; fat 5.8g; sugar 2.2g; salt 0.3g

This is a mixed leaf salad with chicken breast and a Caesar dressing served in a separate pot – a good move, as you could always go without the dressing and save on some of the calories. As it stands, with the dressing, this falls into the medium band for its fat content and has 156 calories per serving – 120 less than the mozzarella and cherry tomato salad.

TOP SWAP TIP

Make your own. The healthiest salads contain some fibre and slower releasing carbohydrates, such as some whole-grain pasta or quinoa (a grain that can be used in the same way as rice), to ensure you have a constant release of energy throughout the afternoon. At home make your own croutons by baking some cubes of bread in the oven.

SWAP ▶ Cheese layered salad

Per 100g (3½oz): calories 165; fat 10.7g; sugar 2.4g; salt 0.4g

Supermarket layered salads tend to consist of some lettuce (usually iceberg) that is 'glued' together with a high-calorie dressing. Added to that it is topped with a layer of Cheddar cheese. With 615 calories per portion and over 10 per cent of its weight from fat, a serving contains almost half an adult woman's daily fat allowance and the equivalent of as much as seven Cadbury's cream eggs. It also has almost one-third the daily intake for salt, so all in all it is not a wise move.

FOR ▶ Prawn layered salad

Per 100g (3½oz): calories 135; fat 7.3g; sugar 2.5g; salt 0.5g

With less fat and fewer calories (there are 510 per portion), this is a better layered-salad option; nevertheless it has 7.3 per cent fat, so not exactly as low-fat as a salad could be. Much of the saving comes from the fact that prawns are lower in fat than cheese.

———————

SWAP ▶ Chicken and potato salad

Per 100g (3½oz): calories 149; fat 10.9g; sugar 1.9g; salt 0.5g

This salad sounds balanced, but it actually has more fat than a giant sausage roll and well over one-half a woman's intake in a single portion. Cut out the dressing and you save 21 calories and 7g of fat, but it still comes in at over the acceptable mark.

FOR ▶ Hummus and falafel salad

Per 100g (3½oz): calories 145; fat 7g; sugar 2.1g; salt 0.8g

Falafel, made from ground chickpeas, are usually deep-fried so they are generally to be avoided as a nibbly food. In this case, they certainly add to the fat content of this salad. A portion (which is larger than the salad above) provides 577 calories and more than one-third of the daily salt intake. However, the chickpeas in the hummus and the falafel provide some protein and you save 16g of fat per serving compared to the chicken and potato salad.

———————

SWAP ▸ Honey and mustard chicken pasta salad

Per 100g (3½oz): calories 173; fat 6.2g; sugar 3.5g; salt 0.2g

This is a pasta salad of which 28 per cent of the weight is a creamy honey and mustard dressing providing most of the 21.7g of fat per portion. In total, this contains 604 calories. Best avoided.

FOR ▸ Beetroot salad bowl

Per 100g (3½oz): calories 90; fat 8g; sugar 3.2g; salt 0.25g

This is more like a salad should be, containing mixed leaves (although they are mostly the nutrient-lacking iceberg variety) with 20 per cent cooked beetroot and cherry tomatoes. The only downfall here is the lemon mayo dressing, which means it's in the not-very-healthy middle band for fat. Still, a serving gives you only 206 calories. You could afford to eat it with a bread roll and still save 250 calories or more. The nutrients in the beetroot might help to lower blood pressure and it contains acetylsalicylic acid, which works like aspirin as an anti-inflammatory, so it's worth eating it regularly.

CHAPTER **EIGHT**

.

Ready meals

THERE'S NO DOUBT THAT we are time crunched – we live our lives in a hurry. Ready meals are billed as the solution to the demands of our lifestyles; they are quick, convenient and appear to provide a nutritious meal in the time it takes to open the packet. We swallow this ideal with unending enthusiasm. As our consumption of fresh produce falls, so sales of processed products such as pies, pizzas and ready meals continue to grow. Demand for pre-prepared fare has risen by about 44 per cent in recent years and it is estimated that almost one-third of adults now consume a ready meal more than once a week.

Ethnic meals are particularly popular, and Chinese, Indian and other Asian recipes make up 40 per cent of the chilled ready-made meal market. Clever marketing means our image of these foods has been radically transformed. Whereas they used to be deemed as the unhealthy and lazy option, they have been repositioned as a premium and nutritious indulgence.

Don't be taken in by the packaging

Among the latest ready meals that have been introduced to the vast market are the 'almost-ready meals', those that invite you to 'cook your own', providing the weighed ingredients you need to prepare a 'home-cooked dish'. What could be better than that?

Don't be fooled. Many pre-prepared meals sold as healthy contain far more fat, calories and salt than the standard version you make at home or eat in a restaurant. Even within brands, the values of products can vary enormously. When comparing packets of a premium macaroni cheese from one supermarket with a similar food from its budget range I found the former, which you would imagine to be a better choice, actually contained almost twice as much fat.

In a survey of chilled ready-made meals by Which?, Morrisons' standard beef lasagne had more fat per 100g (3½oz) than its premium version, and Somerfield's Simply Value beef lasagne had less fat than its Healthy Choice beef lasagne. The highest amounts of fat, saturated fat and salt per 100g (3½oz) were all found in cheese and tomato pizzas. What's more, the labelling on these products can be wildly misleading with fancy claims concealing the hidden truth about what they contain.

So concerned are doctors about the less-than-healthy profile of ready meals that, in the UK, the National Institute for Health and Clinical Excellence (NICE) has issued guidance urging the medical profession to work with food makers specifically to produce more healthy ready meals in order to combat the rise in obesity and type-2 diabetes.

To be fair, there are days when we all lack the time to rustle up fresh ingredients and make a truly home-made meal, and some manufacturers have made huge strides forward in cutting salt and fat from their ready meals, which makes them an option occasionally. But consistency is lacking to such an extent that it is impossible to recommend ready meals en masse.

The beauty of home-made

On a more subtle level, if you live your life on ready meals, your palate and imagination become stifled. Even with the new range of 'almost-ready meals', there is a rigidity to the weighed out and pre-chopped ingredients that makes it unlikely you will add some extra garlic or a few more chillies to enhance the flavour as you might if you had shopped for and prepared your own ingredients from scratch.

You will probably notice that this chapter is shorter than many of the others. That's because recommending even the concept of ready meals weighs heavy on the conscience (and, inevitably in most cases, the waistline). There are so many better 'convenience' meals that can be created at home with just a few ingredients and which provide your body with beneficial nutrients.

You can stir-fry fresh vegetables and noodles in a matter of minutes. A version of macaroni cheese can be knocked together in no time using crème fraîche and grated cheese stirred into pasta. You can even put some sausages in the oven and peel and cook some potatoes in about the time it takes to heat up a saltier, fattier, ready-made version of bangers and mash drenched in a sauce that is a salty excuse for gravy.

For every reason there is for buying a ready meal, there are perhaps a dozen reasons why you should not – at least not on a regular basis. In this case, at least, convenience always means compromise.

How the meals below are presented

All the swaps below are based on serving sizes of 400g (14oz). Be aware that many manufacturers provide information per 100g (3½oz) and you will need to calculate the pack total according to its weight. Ready meals vary tremendously in terms of the quality of ingredients used and the fat, salt and sugar content. This section provides average values for meals based on an analysis of those available in major supermarkets. Make sure you check the packaging carefully as the product you purchase could contain far more (or less) of the nutrients and calories listed.

SWAP ▸ Sausage and mash

Per 400g (14oz) serving: calories 500; fat 25g; sugars 5.0g; salt 3.5g

Hidden salt is a common problem with ready meals and this can be a prime offender. Adults are recommended to consume no more than 6g of salt a day, but this dish provides well over half that amount. Much of the salt comes in the gravy served on top of the two pork sausages and mash. If you want to have bangers and mash, make your own meal using fresh ingredients and good-quality sausages that have a high meat content and no additives or preservatives. That way you can cut fat, salt and calories.

FOR ▸ Lancashire hotpot

Per 400g (14oz) serving: calories 420; fat 17g; sugars 0.3g; salt 2.0g

This is a diced lamb dish with gravy that is topped with sliced potatoes. It contains very little sugar and 4 per cent fat, which makes it far more favourable than the bangers and mash.

SWAP ▶ Chicken and bacon pasta bake

Per 400g (14oz) serving: calories 683; fat 24.8g; sugars 4.8g; salt 2.0g

This sounds like such a simple and appetising dish – penne pasta with 'tender chicken breast', but the fact that it is 'topped with a creamy cheese sauce, smoked bacon and Cheddar cheese' turns it into a healthy-eating nightmare. It is high in calories, total fat (35 per cent of the GDA) and saturated fat (66 per cent of the GDA). Salt levels are better than some, but still too high. Pasta can be so much healthier when served with a freshly made tomato sauce and topped with a sprinkling of cheese.

FOR ▶ Fish pie

Per 400g (14oz) serving: calories 399; fat 12.7g; sugars 4.4g; salt 2.4g

This is a fish pie with haddock in a cheese sauce topped with mashed potato, and you can find healthier versions, like this one, in some of the supermarket ranges, such as Asda. It's not all good news as it is not particularly low in fat and contains too much salt. You'd be much better off making this at home or serving haddock with potatoes and fresh vegetables. Still, you do save considerably on fat and calories compared with the pasta bake.

————

SWAP ▶ Lamb moussaka

Per 400g (14oz) serving: calories 600; fat 40.0g; sugars 6.1g; salt 3g

If ever there was an example of how bad some ready meals can get, this is it. It provides one-third of a woman's daily calories, but a colossal 89 per cent of the maximum amount of saturated fat and 60 per cent of the overall fat she is supposed to consume in a day. It is also high in salt, containing half the daily amount. All of this in one meal.

FOR ▸ Chicken in red wine sauce

Per 400g (14oz) serving: calories 324; fat 3.4g; sugars 8.6g; salt 1.3g

For almost half the calories, you can switch to this meal, which comprises chicken breast in a red wine sauce served with garlic potatoes. It is low in calories and fat. Scan the packaging and you will probably find that the chicken has water added – hardly as nutritionally beneficial as a home-cooked dish. But relatively speaking not a bad choice if served with fresh vegetables.

————

SWAP ▸ Chicken korma

Per 400g (14oz) serving: calories 610; fat 38.2g; sugars 13.3g; salt 2.3g

Chicken korma is made with a creamy sauce that, in this case, contains yoghurt, single cream and coconut milk. The result is a curry that contains more than half a woman's daily fat intake and more than one-third of an adult's salt intake. Bear in mind that you would add rice and 100 or so more calories to this dish.

FOR ▸ Indian dhal vegetable pot

Per 400g (14oz) serving: calories 319; fat 9.9g; sugars 6.5g; salt 1.8g

This individual vegetable curry is low in fat, saturated fat and sugar and has only a medium salt content. Made with cauliflower, chickpeas and fresh spinach, it is high in fibre with 20.1g a pot – that's 84 per cent of the GDA. It is low in saturated fat and salt and also contains fewer calories than many other ready meals. Yet with the pulses and vegetables it contains it is likely to be filling and will give you three of your five daily portions of vegetables. It contains almost half the calories of the korma.

––––––––––

SWAP ▸ Microwaveable cheeseburger

Per 400g (14oz) serving: calories 575; fat 30g; sugars 4.6g; salt 1.1g

This is a microwaveable quarter-pounder burger (often made with just 75 per cent beef with textured soya protein added for bulk). The burger is topped with a slice of processed cheese inside a sesame seed bun and contains a lot of calories for its size (it weighs only 205g so is a small serving). Since it's unlikely you would eat it on its own, the actual amount you consume in a sitting might be even higher. Add chips and it would be close to 900 calories. About 15 per cent of the meal is fat and the serving provides one-third of a man's daily fat requirement.

FOR ▸ Vegetarian chilli

Per 400g (14oz) serving: calories 415; fat 14.6g; sugars 12.0g; salt 1.6g

If it's a light meal that can be bunged in the microwave that you are after, then this is a better bet. It contains tomatoes, rice, 12 per cent sweet potato and onion which, combined, mean there is a decent amount of fibre and vitamin C. It's not too high in fat (3.7 per cent), is low in sugar and saves 150 calories compared to the burger.

SWAP ▶ Chicken arrabiatta

Per 400g (14oz) serving: calories 488; fat 8.7g; sugars 9.9g; salt 1.3g

A pasta dish containing chicken breast and a creamy tomato sauce made with cream and sugar that constitutes a hefty 52 per cent of the product's weight. It is on the medium band for its fat and sugar contents, but contains acceptable levels for salt. Nevertheless, you could do better.

FOR ▶ Mediterranean chicken breasts

Per 400g (14oz) serving: calories 208; fat 5.1g; sugars 3.8g; salt 0.7g

A pack consists of two chicken breasts in a tomato sauce with onions, peppers and feta cheese, although a serving size is half this amount. The product has healthy levels of fat, sugar and salt – a rarity in the ready-meal stakes. Serve with a green salad and a healthy grain – wholegrain rice or quinoa – and you have a balanced meal.

––––––––––

SWAP ▶ Tagliatelle carbonara

Per 400g (14oz) serving: calories 797; fat 41.9g; sugars 4.9g; salt 3.11g

This consists of egg pasta in a creamy cheese sauce topped with mushrooms, pancetta and more cheese. Eat the whole 400g (14oz) pack (half the pack is unlikely to fill you up), and the amount of salt, calories and fat you would consume would be horrendous. It provides well over half a woman's daily fat intake, and more than half an adult's salt intake.

FOR ▶ A healthy-eating-range pasta with a creamy sauce, ham and mushrooms

Per 400g (14oz) serving: calories 361; fat 4.6g; sugars 5.1g; salt 2.37g

There are quite a few savings with this swap to a pasta dish from a supermarket healthy-eating range, especially considering this is the same 400g (14oz) serving size as the carbonara: less than half the calories and one-tenth of the fat are present in this equivalent. Here, the creamy sauce is made with semi-skimmed milk and water, which cuts the amount of fat used. The downsides are the salt it provides per portion (over one-third of an adult's maximum intake) and the fact that the ham used is 'reformed' and made from only 85 per cent meat with water, salt, brown sugar and stabilisers added.

TOP SWAP TIP

What is the best way to buy ready meals?

• Check that there are no additives, preservatives and colourings. The shorter the list of ingredients the better.

• Ideally, salt content should not exceed 2g per portion. Remember, the daily maximum for an adult is 6g.

• Scrutinise labels: healthy-eating ranges are usually lower in fat and calories than standard versions, but not always.

• Premium brands are often the worst offenders in terms of added ingredients like cream and fat.

▶

- Select meals with packaging that has a clear window allowing you to see what's inside. That way you can check to see if there are vegetables or if the food is swimming in a sauce. Choose the former.

- Don't be wooed by claims such as 'nutritionally balanced' and 'healthy eating' that are commonly used to describe ready meals. They mean nothing.

SWAP ▶ Spicy 'jerk' chicken with rice and peas

Per 400g (14oz) serving: calories 640; fat 21.6g; sugars 17.2g; salt 1.9g

This healthy-looking meal consists of 43 per cent cooked white rice and pulses served with chicken thighs marinated in a spicy tomato-based sauce. However, there are few vegetables and the sauce is highly sweetened. Overall it provides 35 per cent of an adult's daily fat requirement and one-third of the daily salt. Better to marinate your own chicken with a spicy piri piri-style sauce and serve with brown rice.

FOR ▶ Chicken and prawn paella

Per 400g (14oz) serving: calories 330; fat 7.0g; sugars 5.4g; salt 1.4g

A slightly smaller serving size than the jerk chicken – this is 300g (10½oz) – yet even taking that into account it is a better choice. It is made with rice, tomatoes, chicken, prawns and peas but it is low in both fat and sugars and saves you 310 calories per portion.

CHAPTER **NINE**

·

Snacking

HOW WE LOVE TO SNACK. Whereas we used to sit down to three square meals a day, our lifestyles now dictate that snacks that are eaten in place of regular meals contribute a huge amount to our total calorie intake. We consume 15 per cent more snack foods than we did ten years ago, and the variety available to us seems to increase by the week.

In itself, the concept of snacking is not unhealthy. Topping up blood sugar and energy levels with smaller, more regular mini-meals is a balanced approach to eating. What matters is what we are snacking on. Fresh fruit and vegetable crudités are not going to cause many inches to be gained around the waistline even if we eat them by the plate load. But, instead, we consume snack foods that are high in fat, sugar and salt often without realising it.

Psychologists have found that some people do feel guilty about their snacking habit. Research at Tufts University revealed that 33 per cent of people snack only when nobody is watching, and half feel guilty after a snack treat. On average, the results showed that 50 per cent of people admit they can't go a full day without having at least one snack between meals. Crisps were the most popular choice, followed by chocolates, biscuits and cakes. What is lurking in some snacks might surprise you.

Crisps

Our all-time favourite savoury snack food: crisps. They may be fried in fat and smothered in salt, but that doesn't deter us. On average, each adult consumes about 150 packets of them a year. Even if you don't describe yourself as a crisp fan, the likelihood is that you have a favourite flavour; favourites have rarely changed much over the years despite more than 100 varieties now being available. Cheese and onion take the top spot, followed by ready salted, salt and vinegar, prawn cocktail and chicken.

When you consider how many packs of fried potato slices we eat, you do wonder what effect the habit is having on our health. In fact, the consequences are unlikely to be good. A few years ago, the British Heart Foundation (BHF) launched a major campaign that warned that half of all British children were, in effect, drinking 5 litres (8¾ pints) of cooking oil a year by virtue of their packet-a-day habit, with crisps being placed in 69 per cent of lunchboxes. Soaring rates of obesity and type-2 diabetes were, the BHF warned, the likely side effects of a lifelong crisp habit. Indeed, crisps were named as the food most closely linked to weight gain in a large study of American people's diets that was published in the *New England Journal of Medicine*.

The slightly healthier choices

Overall, there have been reductions in salt, fat and sugar content, and most crisps now contain up to 80 per cent less saturated fat and 55 per cent less salt than they did ten years ago. And there are healthier options to the standard potato crisp now available. Kettle chips – a relatively new arrival having first gone on sale in the 1990s – are billed as better for you, and their irregular, crunchy appearance along with their higher price certainly suggests they are. Like their down-market counterparts, kettle chips are still cooked in vegetable oil which is not the healthiest to cook with as it is unstable at high temperatures and prone to chemical changes that oxidise fat and can raise cholesterol levels. They are also (mostly) sprinkled with salt, but generally they don't contain any monosodium glutamate (MSG), colours or flavours and do have among the lowest calorie and fat contents per 100g (3½oz). Baked crisps are similarly less harmful to the waistline with up to 70 per cent less total fat than standard crisps.

Not that this means a green light for consumption. Far from it. About one-third of the weight of a regular bag (25g/1oz) of crisps is fat compared to the 0.1mg of fat you would find in boiled potatoes. Typically, the salt content of crisps is about 1.9g per 100g (3½oz) whereas potatoes contain virtually none. Most crisps contain artificial flavourings, MSG and acidity regulators that combine to trick the palate into thinking you want to consume more. It's hardly surprising then that crisps are a hard habit to break. We may love them but ideally, they are best limited to an occasional pack or avoided altogether. If you must indulge, select the healthiest of the fried potato crop. Values for each swap below are per 100g (3½oz); a regular crisp packet is 25g (1oz) in size.

SWAP ▶ McCoy's ridge-cut salt and malt vinegar

Per 100g (3½oz): calories 516; fat 30.6g; sugar 1.0g; salt 2.6g

The ridged surface means that these crisps grab onto more of the sunflower oil. They also have added MSG and acidity regulators.

FOR ▶ Kettle chips sea salt and balsamic vinegar

Per 100g (3½oz): calories 502; fat 28.4g; sugar 1.3g; salt 1.9g

A saving of a couple of grams of fat per 100g (3½oz) but, more importantly, these contain more fibre than many crisps (6.1 per cent compared to an average 1.2 per cent in many others) and no artificial flavourings or MSG. Seasonings are from sea salt and balsamic vinegar, although sugar is also added.

TOP SWAP TIP

Opt for small bags. Sales of bigger bags of so-called 'sharing' crisps designed for sociable consumption are rising, and portion sizes have generally increased by about 30 per cent in recent years. But be careful, because once you open a big bag (even if you are sharing it with the family), you are likely to eat more than you would if you had a regular 25g (1oz) bag of crisps.

SWAP ▶ Walkers prawn cocktail quavers

Per 100g (3½oz): calories 537; fat 31g; sugar 1.7g; salt 2.11g

Made with potato starch and sunflower oil mixed together with MSG, salt, artificial sweeteners, rice flour and dried onion powder among other ingredients, these are among the highest in fat and calories on a weight-for-weight basis. Because there are fewer of them in a bag – it only weighs 16g (½oz) – the manufacturers make much of the fact that a serving provides only 88 calories. Don't be misled into thinking they are in fact low in fat.

FOR ▶ KP hula hoops

Per 100g (3½oz): calories 514; fat 28.4g; sugar 0.4g; salt 2.3g

These are made from an unappetising-sounding mixture of potato starch, dried potato, rice and maize flour and then shaped into the characteristic hoops. With 129 calories per 25g (1oz) bag, they are by no means a healthy snack, but do offer a saving compared to quavers.

TOP SWAP TIP

Following a few guidelines will help you to choose the least unhealthy crisps:

- Crinkle crisps with a ridged surface tend to have the highest fat count, as more fat is required to coat the cut surface of the potato.

- Stronger flavours can mean higher sugar contents, so stick to the plain variety.

- Don't assume that 'posh' crisps or 'light' crisps are a healthier choice. Many are not. In fact, value brands often offer a product that is nutritionally similar to many of the so-called healthier choice crisps.

- Look for packs that contain no MSG or artificial flavourings. They do exist.

SWAP ▶ Walkers ready salted

Per 100g (3½oz): calories 537; fat 34.1g; sugar 0.4g;
salt 1.52g

These gain a plus point for containing only three ingredients
(potatoes, oil and salt), but lose several for their fat and salt
content, both of which are high.

FOR ▶ Walkers baked ready salted

Per 100g (3½oz): calories 401; fat 8g; sugar 6.5g;
salt 1.52g

Here you get a saving of 136 calories per 100g (3½oz) because
of the production method; these are baked in oil, not fried.
Unfortunately, sugar, starch, oil and emulsifiers are added to
make them as crisp as the original. And they are still high in
salt, so only eat them occasionally.

TOP SWAP TIP

Be careful how you dip. Dips are considered healthy
options and have become a regular accompaniment to
crisps for many. But dips such as hummus, taramasalata
and blue cheese can be high in fat and calories. A survey
conducted by the World Cancer Research Fund showed
that two-thirds of people underestimate the number of
calories in chickpea and oil-based hummus. On average it
contains 332 calories per 100g (3½oz) – the same amount
of calories as found in a chocolate brownie. If you want to
dip, the best swap is a tomato-based salsa, which is low in

▶

calories – 78 per 100g (3½oz) – and fat (4 per cent). The tomatoes provide some of the pigment lycopene that can help to protect the skin from sun damage, among other health benefits. Tatziki, made from yoghurt, is also up there on the favourable swaps and is high in calcium, but low in calories – 66 per 100g (3½oz). Limit the amount of creamy dips, such as blue cheese, and sour cream and chives, as they tend to contain 30 per cent fat and 300 calories or more per 100g (3½oz). Likewise, taramasalata – made from cod roe, oil and breadcrumbs – because almost half its weight is fat and it contains close to 500 calories per 100g (3½oz). That's before you dip anything in it.

SWAP ▶ Walkers salt and vinegar chipsticks

Per 100g (3½oz): calories 481; fat 23g; sugar 0.6g; salt 3.68g

Made from maize, vegetable oils and potato granules, with MSG and preservatives, these are as far removed from a traditional crisp as you could get. They also contain very high salt levels.

FOR ▶ Skips prawn cocktail

Per 100g (3½oz): calories 344; fat 4.7g; sugar 1.1g; salt 0.4g

Like chipsticks, skips haven't been near a real potato and are made instead with tapioca starch and maize flour. If you are partial to a 'synthetic' crisp taste, then at least they save you 140 calories per 100g (3½oz), contain less than one-quarter of the fat and reach only the medium level for salt (not bad in the crisp world).

IS POPCORN THE HEALTHIEST CHOICE?

Popcorn has been gaining a reputation as a healthy snack ever since Madonna claimed to have lost weight eating it between meals in the 1990s. Now, though, there is scientific, and not just celebrity backing, to its claims to be good for you. Somewhat surprisingly, scientists reporting to the American Chemical Society found that it contains more of the healthful antioxidant substances called poly-phenols than are found in fruits and vegetables. This is because the polyphenols in popcorn are more concentrated. Popcorn contains only about 4 per cent water, whereas fruits and vegetables are made up of 90 per cent water. The polyphenols contained in the fruits and vegetables are diluted compared to the popcorn. Weight for weight, then, popcorn contains more. That piece of popcorn shell that gets stuck in your teeth is called the 'hull' and it actually packs the highest concentration of antioxidants and fibre, which may make you think twice the next time you're tempted to spit it out. As the only popular snack that is 100 per cent unprocessed whole grain, popcorn gains other nutritional points.

The good, the bad ...

Of course, not all popcorn is good. Scientists studying its benefits are referring only to plain, air-popped popcorn, not the toffee- or butter-drenched varieties that are no better for you than sweets or crisps. Air-popped popcorn has the lowest number of calories: 387 per 100g (3½oz), or 31

➤

per decent-sized serving. Microwave popcorn has twice as many: about 43 per cent of microwave popcorn is fat compared to 28 per cent if you pop the corn in oil yourself; and if you pop your own with butter or oil, this also has double the amount as air-popped popcorn.

A 200g (7oz) bag of Butterkist toffee popcorn contains a whopping 830 calories and is 10 per cent fat. At the cinema, a large bag of sweet popcorn could contain an alarming 1,800 calories – the equivalent of a large curry with sides and two bottles of beer. A large bag of salted popcorn contains about 1,779 calories – the same as a three-course meal of pizza, garlic bread and trifle. If plain popcorn is too bland, try adding low-calorie flavourings such as chilli powder, cinnamon or curry powder. Lightly spraying the popcorn with a touch of water or olive oil can help the spices to stick to the popcorn.

Biscuits

One biscuit is never enough, making biscuits the nibbler's nightmare – once that packet is opened, the sugar, fat and calories can mount up before you know it. Research has shown that the reason we hit the biscuit tin, particularly when we're at work, is more than likely to be boredom. And the average office worker packs away up to one-third of their daily calorie allowance on snacks like biscuits and cookies.

On a weight-for-weight basis, biscuits are high in fat; many contain vegetable oils that have been hardened or hydrogenated (see page 89) and which have been shown to wreak more havoc on our bodies than saturated animal fats such as butter. Biscuits are far from the healthiest snack around and should be limited, especially if you are trying to lose weight. Select wisely though, and you can enjoy your treat – occasionally.

SWAP ▶ Butter shortbread

Per biscuit: calories 95; fat 5.3g; sugars 2.6g; salt 0.1g

On the plus side, butter shortbread contains only flour, butter, sugar and salt, but that mix does make a finger of shortbread pretty high in fat.

FOR ▶ Garibaldi

Per biscuit: calories 40; fat 0.9g; sugars 3.8g; salt trace

Surprisingly low in calories and with not too much fat, these biscuits have the added advantage of some fibre, which is good for promoting a healthy bowel, and other nutrients such as iron (a rarity in many biscuits) from the 38 per cent currants. A good snack – if you can stick to a couple – and it saves you 55 calories per biscuit.

SWAP ▶ Milk chocolate digestive

Per biscuit: calories 85; fat 4.0g; sugars 5.1g; salt 0.2g

A milk chocolate coating on a biscuit bumps up the calorie content by 20 per biscuit and doubles the fat content. Milk chocolate digestives do have some fibre, which will help your digestion. Dark chocolate digestives provide slightly less fat, but it's best to avoid the toppings altogether.

FOR ▸ Digestive

Per biscuit: calories 71; fat 3.1g; sugar 2.5g; salt 0.2g

Better on the calorie, fat and sugar fronts than the chocolate-covered digestive. This is based on an average-sized biscuit, although smaller versions are often sold for biscuits with cheese and would contain fewer calories. It's not all good news. Like many biscuits, digestives are highly sweetened and contain at least one type of sugar. They also contain more salt than many biscuits.

RESIST TEMPTATION AT WORK

Research has shown that the workplace presents ample opportunity for weakening of resolve when it comes to weight loss. We eat 30 per cent more calories in company than we do alone, and women are more likely to be influenced by the diet patterns of colleagues than men. Eating behaviourists at Cornell University found that female secretaries ate 5.6 times more chocolates if the chocolates were placed on a nearby desk than if the secretary had to stand up and walk 2m (around 6ft) to get them. In another experiment they showed that office workers sitting near glass dishes filled with sweets ate 71 per cent more – or 77 calories a day – than those sitting near white, opaque dishes of the same confectionary. Over the course of a year, the clear dish would have added more than 2.25kg (5lb) of extra weight. Here's how to avoid temptation:

• **Keep healthy food in view** You are more likely to eat what you can see, so if someone comes in with cakes

▶

and biscuits, make sure your celery sticks and carrots are within view on your desk.

- **Don't throw away wrappers** Studies have shown that keeping empty chocolate wrappers or crisp bags on your desk can act as a deterrent to eating more; it gives a tangible reminder of what you have previously eaten.

- **Put it away** If the office feeder hands out biscuits and insists you take one, get into the habit of removing it from reach immediately. Put it, unopened, in your bag or lock it away in a drawer.

SWAP ▸ Jammie dodgers

Per biscuit: calories 83; fat 2.8g; sugar 6.8g; salt trace

Twenty-six per cent of the weight of each biscuit contains raspberry jam sweetened with HFCS (see page 196) and sugar. The biscuit itself also contains sugar and golden syrup, which is the reason it is a high-sugar food.

FOR ▸ ginger nuts

Per biscuit: calories 47; fat 1.7g; sugar 3g; salt 0.1g

Ginger nuts comprise almost one-third sugar, and are often sweetened with HFCS (check the label for one that isn't), sugar and molasses, the latter being rich in minerals and they are also a reasonable source of iron. Three ginger nuts supply one-tenth of a woman's intake for iron. Although their ginger content isn't particularly high, some people find they are helpful before a journey or to ease queasiness. Plus, they save you 36 calories per biscuit over the jammie dodgers.

SWAP ▶ Custard creams

Per biscuit: calories 65; fat 2.7g; sugars 3.7g; salt trace

The cream filling is highly sweetened with sugar and synthetic flavours, and this bumps up the total sugar content to 29 per cent of the weight. Overall, however, they don't contain too much fat for a filled biscuit. But you can do better.

FOR ▶ Fig roll

Per biscuit: calories 64; fat 1.4g; sugar 5.5g; salt trace

It's not so much what you are losing here in terms of calories, but what you are gaining elsewhere. Fig rolls contain half the fat of even reduced-fat biscuits and no hydrogenated vegetable oil. The fig paste they contain provides sugar but also 15 per cent of the daily minimum intake of fibre.

––––––––––

SWAP ▶ Malted milk

Per biscuit: calories 44; fat 1.9g; sugar 1.4g; salt trace

Malted milk biscuits contain dried whole milk and are sweetened with sugar and glucose syrup. On the whole, they are not too bad a choice, but you can do better when it comes to a dunking favourite.

FOR ▶ Rich tea

Per biscuit: calories 38; fat 1.3g; sugar 1.7g; salt trace

A plain biscuit with very little fat – they are lower even than reduced-fat digestives and have 30 fewer calories. There are 6 fewer than the malted milk. Less encouraging is that they contain hydrogenated fats, sugar and HFCS – so really an occasional treat.

SWAP ▸ Bourbon

Per biscuit: calories 70; fat 3.0g; sugar 4.3g; salt trace

Chocolate bourbons are highly sweetened with sugar, dextrose and glucose syrup. They also contain hydrogenated vegetable fat, unless it states otherwise on the packet. They are not the highest calorie biscuit around, but are far from the lowest.

FOR ▸ Jaffa cake

Per biscuit: calories 46; fat 1.0g; sugar 6.4g; salt trace

Containing only 8 per cent fat – very low for a chocolate-covered biscuit – jaffa cakes are a firm favourite among athletes and sporty types. Each biscuit has 24 fewer calories than a bourbon. They have a fairly high sugar content – almost one teaspoon per biscuit – but are free from hydrogenated fats and contain virtually no salt.

BEWARE THE DEVIL'S CANDY

High fructose corn syrup (HFCS) – also sometimes called glucose fructose syrup, glucose corn syrup and medium fructose corn syrup – is an intense sweetener. It is used in a vast and diverse array of food products, and has been labelled 'the Devil's candy' by some scientists. You won't find bottles of this stuff on supermarket shelves next to other sugary syrups, but scan the ingredients' lists on everything from cola and iced tea to biscuits, chocolate bars and cakes, and it is likely to be lurking among the additives. It is ubiquitous in our food supplies.

▶

Reports suggest the average person now consumes about 200 calories a day from HFCS – that's 12 teaspoons – an increase from 2 calories a day in 1970, and about a tenth of the advised daily calorific intake depending on your sex. And there are concerns that it's too much. Indeed, eminent scientists have suggested that it is the rising intake of HFCS that is directly fuelling the spiralling obesity problem. A paper in the *American Journal of Clinical Nutrition* supplied statistics correlating a rise in obesity to a rise in HFCS consumption. All of this may be coincidence. Alternatively, is there something more insidious about this sweetener that is short-wiring our metabolism to make us fat?

A not very natural product

A distant derivative of corn, HFCS starts off as maize starch. It is converted to glucose, which is then converted to fructose. Manufacturers, mostly based in the US corn belt, are fighting against demonisation of the sweetener, claiming the product is natural because it is made from corn and contains no additives or colourings. But this is more sci-fi than home cooking. Corn kernels are first placed in stainless steel vats and spun at high velocity before three enzymes are added to trigger 'molecular rearrangements'. These enzymes turn most of the glucose molecules in corn into fructose, which makes the substance sweeter. At 90 per cent fructose, the syrup mixture is mixed with corn syrup (100 per cent glucose molecules) to get the right mix of fructose and glucose.

►

The end product is a clear, gloopy liquid that is considerably sweeter than sugar. Unlike many manufactured sweeteners, such as aspartame and saccharin, however, it is not low in calories, containing about the same number as normal sugar (25 in a heaped teaspoon). Studies have indicated that the body metabolises fructose, the sweetest of natural sugars, in a way that may promote weight gain. Specifically, fructose does not trigger the release of the hormones that help to regulate appetite and fat storage, nor does it stimulate insulin and leptin (hormones that help to dampen appetite).

Why is it used instead of sugar?

Cost was the main reason that manufacturers switched from using cane and beet sugar to the corn-based sweetener three decades ago. HFCS is used so widely simply because it is cheap to produce. It just gives manufacturers more sweetness for their buck. It has become ubiquitous in our food supply and the reasons for using it are increasingly diverse. It is easier to blend into liquids and keeps its sweetness better than sugar, so it is added to many soft drinks, including Pepsi and Coke.

HFCS helps to prevent freezer-burn of food and reduces crystallisation, so it's used in a lot of frozen products, such as ice-cream. It turns baked products brown and keeps them soft when cooked, so you will find it in many cakes, pastries and bread rolls, crackers and breakfast cereals. A can of cola or lemonade can contain as much as 13 teaspoons of sugar in the form of HFCS; a low-fat, fruit-flavoured yoghurt

►

can conceal 10 teaspoons of the fructose-based sweetener in one pot. Many over-the-counter cough and cold medications contain it, as do some pickled meats and pizzas. It is increasingly difficult to avoid HFCS but the message is to scan labels and limit it where you can, avoid buying too many ready-made meals, cakes and biscuits and prepare home-cooked food whenever possible to avoid it.

Chocolate

Our guilty pleasure: chocolate. There is nothing quite like the velvety melt of chocolate on the tongue to tease the palate and tempt our taste buds. The good news is that, if you stick to the dark variety in small amounts, chocolate is good for you. Dark chocolate is a useful source of iron, and all chocolate supplies the mineral potassium. Due in part to the presence of a substance called phenylethylamine (PEA), which occurs naturally in the brain, eating chocolate can also have an uplifting effect on your mood while the stimulants theobromine and caffeine that it contains can increase alertness.

That's not all. Over the past two decades scientists have unearthed many more potent health benefits for the cocoa bean. Studies have shown that it is rich in flavonoids: powerful natural antioxidants that destroy the harmful molecules known as free radicals that can circulate in our bodies, raising the risk of disease. Dark chocolate has been linked to the control of high blood pressure and heart disease, and even bowel cancer. One particular plant compound in chocolate, called epicatechin, seems to stimulate the same response in muscles as vigorous activity. It could even be that chocolate helps with age-related muscle loss.

Milk and white are not the same as dark

Spanish scientists showed the antioxidant compounds in dark chocolate seem to help the body use its insulin more effectively to control blood sugar levels. As a result, blood sugar levels are lowered and diabetes risks are reduced. Milk and white chocolate do not share the same benefits. While milk chocolate contains some minerals, they are in much diluted concentrations compared to those present in dark chocolate. White chocolate, which contains no cocoa, has been shown to make skin blood flow slow down – a sign that blood vessels are functioning below par. It would also seem to raise blood cholesterol levels whereas dark chocolate kept them in check.

Even more welcoming – if remarkable – is that people who indulge in dark chocolate regularly tend to stay slimmer. A study published in the *Journal of the Archives of Internal Medicine* showed that of 1,000 people, those who ate dark chocolate a few times a week were slimmer than those who ate very little. It might be loaded with calories, but scientists think the ingredients may encourage weight loss rather than fat synthesis.

Even for the dark stuff it's not all good news, however. A small 125g (4½oz) bar of dark chocolate contains as much caffeine as a cup of instant coffee. And, its average 30 per cent fat content means chocolate contains about 500 calories per 100g (3½oz). Very sugary bars, such as milk chocolate fondant or toffee fillings, are more likely to cause tooth decay and weight gain than offset any health problems.

Size matters

Manufacturers are also 'super-sizing' many popular milk chocolate bars so that they provide even more sugar, calories and fat per serving. For health benefits, only dark chocolate reigns supreme. But if you fancy a nibble of the sweet stuff, it's a chocolate minefield out there. All values are per 100g (3½oz) of chocolate.

SWAP ▸ Green & Black's organic white chocolate

Per 100g (3½oz): calories 580; fat 38.2g; sugars 51.3g; salt 0.2g

This bar may use high-quality organic ingredients but white chocolate offers none of the benefits of dark chocolate in terms of the vitamins and minerals they provide. There is some calcium, but really it's just a sugary treat.

FOR ▸ Green & Black's organic 70% cocoa chocolate

Per 100g (3½oz): calories 575; fat 41.6g; sugars 28.9g; salt 0.13g

Despite its health benefits in terms of antioxidants, don't mistake dark chocolate for being particularly low in calories. Generally, it contains more calories and fat than milk chocolate and, in this case, a higher total fat content than white. Still, it is worth the switch. You save minimal calories, but gain disease-fighting benefits if you consume around 4 squares a day.

––––––––––

SWAP ▸ Cadbury's dairy milk

Per 100g (3½oz): calories 530; fat 29.8g; sugars 56.7g; salt 0.23g

Cadbury's make much of the fact that dairy milk is made with fresh milk as opposed to the milk powder in many other bars; however, it is not a particularly good option on the calorie front. Eat five chunks of dairy milk and you get about 165 calories.

FOR ▸ Galaxy caramel

Per 100g (3½oz): calories 480; fat 27.0g; sugars 56g; salt 0.3g

This gooey, caramel-filled milk chocolate bar contains glucose syrup as well as sugar, yet still has less sugar (and fat) than dairy milk. Not something that should be eaten regularly, as the stickiness will cling to your teeth and is likely to cause tooth decay. As an occasional treat, it saves 50 calories per 100g (3½oz). A small 48g (1½oz) bar contains 239 calories.

SWAP ▸ Snickers

Per 100g (3½oz): calories 511; fat 28.4g; sugar 54.5g; salt 0.2g

An average 58g (2oz) bar of snickers – containing nougat, caramel, peanuts and milk chocolate – contains 296 calories. Its fat levels are lower than some chocolate bars, but you can do better. The good news is that the maker of snickers, Mars, have announced plans to stop selling chocolate products containing more than 250 calories by the end of 2013. Mars has also said it will reduce sodium levels in all its products by 25 per cent by 2015. For now, though, this bar is worth swapping.

FOR ▸ Cadbury's fruit and nut

Per 100g (3½oz): calories 482; fat 26g; sugar 54g; salt 0.24g

If it's the nutty bars you like, this swap saves you 29 calories per 100g (3½oz) and, although the average bar is smaller in size – 48g (1½oz) – it also saves you 56 calories per bar. Unfortunately, the fruit and nut content is not very high and you would need to eat a lot of the bars to gain health benefits such as added fibre, and that would, of course, mean a lot more calories.

SWAP ▶ Nestlé after eights

Per 100g (3½oz): calories 432; fat 11g; sugar 66g; salt trace

The favourite after-dinner mint consists of dark chocolate with a peppermint fondant filling containing sugar and glucose syrup. There are 35 calories per sweet and it is easy to consume 4–6 before you know it. That would be almost 200 calories.

FOR ▶ Fry's chocolate cream

Per 100g (3½oz): calories 410; fat 13g; sugar 64.8g; salt trace

There is more fondant filling than chocolate in this bar (53 per cent of the weight), which reduces the calories compared to a straight chocolate bar and also compared to after eights. It's not all good news; the sticky, sweet fondant is not good for teeth so shouldn't be eaten too often. With 210 calories per 50g (1¾oz) bar, though, it's not a bad choice calorie-wise.

––––––––––

SWAP ▶ Cadbury's crunchie

Per 100g (3½oz): calories 465; fat 18.9g; sugar 69.5g; salt trace

Crunchie bars are honeycomb covered with a relatively thin layer of milk chocolate which keeps their fat content low but makes them particularly high in sugar.

FOR ▶ Mars bar

Per 100g (3½oz): calories 446; fat 17.4g; sugar 68.3g; salt trace

Weight for weight a Mars bar contains fewer calories overall than a crunchie and is probably a bit more filling, but be careful: the bar sizes differ, so whereas you get 185 calories in a 40g (1½oz) crunchie, you get 260 calories in a standard 58g (2oz)

Mars bar (reduced in size from 62.5g (2⅛oz) a few years ago).
Have a snack-size Mars bar – 38g (1¼oz) – and you have 190
calories. If Mars stick to their promise, none of their chocolate
bars will contain more than 250 calories in the next few years,
making their best-seller a safer bet.

WHAT THE CHOCOLATE TERMS MEAN

- **Milk chocolate** Anything labelled milk chocolate must
  contain at least 20 per cent cocoa solids as well as
  cocoa butter. Vegetable fat is often added, although
  the better milk chocolates contain none.

- **Dark chocolate** Any plain or dark chocolate should
  contain at least 35 per cent cocoa solids. Some
  varieties of chocolate contain 55–70 per cent cocoa
  solids. Chocolate connoisseurs enjoy 85 per cent and
  even 100 per cent cocoa solids, but at that level a bar
  can begin to taste bitter.

- **White chocolate** is a bit of a misnomer because it
  contains no cocoa solids at all and many consider it
  not to be 'proper' chocolate. It does, however, contain
  cocoa butter. Cheaper brands contain vegetable fats.

Cakes

It's difficult to think of something harder to resist than a rich,
moist, freshly home-baked cake. Given their basic ingredients –
flour, eggs, butter and sugar – even home-made cakes are always

high in sugar and most contain moderate to high amounts of fat. That mix is what makes a home-made cake so delicious, and the effort taken to make your own is well worth the outcome.

With ready-made cakes, what you get is less straightforward. Other ingredients are thrown in that alter the taste and distort the sugar and fat content. On most labels you will see dried pasteurised egg, invert sugar syrup and sometimes glucose syrup as staple ingredients. Preservatives and flavourings are often added to give it a chemically induced home-made flavour. And many are also a source of harmful trans-fats, the result of oils being hardened by a chemical process, and which are linked to raised cholesterol levels. In every case, it is better to make your own, but there are some surprising savings to be made if you do take a detour down the cake aisle at the supermarket. Values are per cake or slice of cake.

SWAP ▶ Krispy Crème butterscotch fudge doughnut

Per cake: calories 372; fat 17g; sugar 49g; salt 0.1g

Krispy Crème doughnuts have developed something of a cult following around the world with people clamouring to try their signature glazed and cream-filled fare. The calorie content of this doughnut is the equivalent, for example, of a bowl of gazpacho and a serving of sirloin steak, new potatoes and two veg, with honeydew melon to follow. It contains 53 per cent sugar and 18 per cent fat.

FOR ▶ Jam doughnut

Per cake: calories 205; fat 6.9g; sugar 8.5g; salt 0.6g

Who would have thought that a jam doughnut would be considered a better option to anything, since it is a sugar-coated, deep-fried cake. Yet you save 170 calories and 10g of fat with this

indulgence. Even the lowest calorie option from Krispy Crème –
its original glazed – has 217 calories and 25 per cent fat.

————

SWAP ▸ Lemon cupcake

Per cake: calories 252; fat 10.4g; sugar 35g; salt 0.4g

The new generation of cupcakes are often topped with significant amounts of sugar frosting, often sweetened with glucose
syrup and sugar as well as icing sugar. A large cupcake can easily
notch up 400 calories.

FOR ▸ Cherry Bakewell

Per cake: calories 221; fat 9.9g; sugar 20.3g; salt 0.2g

Cherry bakewells tend to be high in sugar and fat, partly due
to their pastry casing and also the almond-flavoured filling. Be
careful, as they can also contain trans-fats, which are linked to
raised cholesterol levels; however, if you like an iced topping,
this swap will save you 35 calories and about 2g of fat per cake.

————

SWAP ▸ Chocolate brownie

Per cake: calories 340; fat 16g; sugar 34g; salt 0.2g

An 80g (2¾oz) brownie typically contains 14 per cent chocolate,
a huge 43 per cent sugar and almost one-fifth of its weight is fat.

FOR ▸ Chocolate mini roll

Per cake: calories 120; fat 5.5g; sugar 13.3g; salt 0.15g

The vanilla-flavoured filling made with glucose syrup and sugar
is almost one-fifth of the mini roll's weight. It is very high in

sugar (46 per cent) but its small size keeps the calories down, so that there are over 200 fewer than in the brownie.

––––––––

SWAP ▶ Carrot cake

Per 72g (2½oz) slice: calories 265; fat 12g; sugar 21g; salt 0.4g

The 21 per cent cream cheese frosting in this carrot cake adds fat, as does the centre layer of buttercream. Both are sweetened. Don't think the carrots make up for this nutritional downfall – only one-tenth of the cake comprises grated carrot. Other ingredients include pasteurised egg and dried glucose syrup. It also has an unhealthy level of salt.

FOR ▶ Victoria sponge

Per 75g (2¾oz) slice: calories 250; fat 12g; sugar 19g; salt 0.3g

It's hard to believe that a slice of this jam and buttercream-filled cake is better on the calorie front than the healthy-sounding carrot cake, but it does contain slightly fewer calories and less sugar. Not a big saving, but every calorie counts.

––––––––

SWAP ▶ Iced fruit cake

Per 75g (2¾oz) slice: calories 205; fat 5g; sugar 26g; salt 0.1g

Fruit cake tends not to be too high in fat – typically about 6–8 per cent of its weight. The mix of dried fruit – raisins, currants, glacé cherries, mixed candied peel – adds a little fibre and some iron, but many are over-sweetened with molasses, syrups and sugar. Typically, half the weight is from sugars (the dried fruit also contributes).

FOR ▶ Fruit malt loaf

Per 35g (1¼oz) slice: calories 85; fat 0.6g; sugar 5g; salt 0.2g

This loaf contains 14 per cent raisins, which means it has better iron and fibre levels than many cakes. It contains some sugar, but is low in fat, making it a favourite with active types. The dried fruit also means it is a better source of iron, potassium and fibre than many cakes. You will often find malt loaf handed out for refuelling to athletes who have completed marathons or triathlons and it is also used by walkers. A worthy swap indeed, but more particularly if you are active.

––––––––

SWAP ▶ Battenburg cake

Per 65g (2¼oz) slice: calories 157; fat 5g; sugar 21g; salt 0.2g

The Battenburg is a sponge cake covered with apricot jam and almond paste (which accounts for almost half its weight). It's high in sugar but some brands do use free-range eggs and no hydrogenated fat.

FOR ▶ Madeira cake

Per 35g/1¼oz slice: calories 147; fat 5.7g; sugar 11.7g; salt 0.2g

A classic Madeira cake contains about 20 per cent butter and so very little (if any) trans-fats. It's a plain cake so no need for large amounts of colourings and flavourings. And it saves you 10 calories and 10g of sugar per slice compared to the Battenburg.

The benefits of home-cooked food

Unsurprisingly, the consequences of these lifestyle changes are dire. Poor dietary habits combined with a lack of physical activity means that one in three children in the UK who leaves primary school is now either obese or overweight. What is known is that significant changes needn't be expensive or time-consuming. Restoring traditional values such as reverting to simple, home-cooked food could go a long way to stemming these problems. Research has shown that children from homes where the family regularly gathers around the table tend to eat more fruit and vegetables than those from homes where mealtimes are not a central focus of the day. There's also plenty of evidence that these children are less overweight or obese and consume more fibre, calcium and vitamins. Likewise, their consumption of junk and fast food, including soft drinks and takeaways, is lower.

There are subtle psychological reasons why a family meal is better, too. Parents who make sure the family sits down together for a communal meal are more likely to provide healthier food. Children who eat these meals grow up in a culture of enjoying mealtimes and learn to understand that healthier food is good for them and to enjoy it. By talking with the family at mealtimes, children (and parents) have been shown to slow down the rate at which they eat and consume fewer calories than those who eat their meals in front of the television. And you don't have to follow the complex recipes set down by a celebrity chef. Meals can be simple and require the least culinary skill imaginable to set your children on the path to better health. Pasta with a fresh tomato sauce, baked fish with vegetables, a jacket potato, omelettes and home-made pizza topped with vegetables are all true convenience foods that can be prepared quickly and have none of the hidden ingredients that food manufacturers ply their products with.

The difficulties with buying ready meals for children

This brings me to another sticking point. As parents' lifestyles have become more time-crunched, so the market for ready meals specifically marketed for children and as an alternative to home cooking for busy mums has soared. Most supermarkets now produce their own ranges of pre-prepared children's meals that are sold alongside specialist brands that purportedly offer high-quality, organic and well-balanced ingredients that meet the nutritional needs of a young diet. These products are best avoided. Many contain levels of salt and sugar that are way too high to be considered healthy for youngsters. As a result, the dishes may be training the palates of youngsters to enjoy ingredients that can contribute to poor health in later life.

Scan the labels, and it's not difficult to find products aimed at children that have a worse nutritional profile than the equivalent adult version. In one survey, a children's range of beef lasagne was found to be laced with 5.4g of sugar per 100g (3½oz) of its weight – double the amount in a similar product for adults. The same ready meal contains 1g of salt per pack – half the entire daily recommended maximum for a child aged one to three.

More than any other sector of the food market, children's food has become over-complicated and confusing to the point that parents are now unsure what they are buying. It is an area where good food swapping is crucial. There is no doubt that eating healthy, nutritious food sets your children up for life. They are less likely to suffer with an expanding waistline and to be at risk of diabetes and heart disease in later life. And they will also thrive in other ways. A good diet is crucial in a child's early life, because the brain grows at its fastest rate during the first three years. Research at the University of Bristol showed that toddlers fed a diet packed with sugars, fat and processed foods had lower IQs than those fed pasta, salad and fruits. They suggested that head growth in the pre-school years is linked to intellectual ability and that good nutrition encourages optimal brain growth.

A good diet helps children academically

It's never too late to start swapping to better choices. Links between diet and academic and athletic ability are in little doubt. Pupils have been shown to achieve lower scores in tests after eating takeaway meals such as burgers and chips more than three times a week even when parental income, race and pupils' weight are taken into account. Some children's scores in literacy and numeracy tests dropped by up to 16 per cent compared to the average when they ate a nutritionally poor diet.

Don't let kids become dieters

It's not just weight problems that are rising among children and adolescents. There has also been a marked increase in concerns about appearance that currently plague adolescents. And that can lead to the unhealthy habit of skipping meals. One survey of 32,000 10 to 15-year-olds by the Schools Health Education Unit in the UK revealed that teenage girls are routinely skipping up to two meals a day. Breakfast is the most common meal forfeited (26 per cent of 14 and 15-year-olds start the day on an empty stomach), but 22 per cent miss lunch and one in ten restrict their food to one daily meal. What has caused this mass shift towards a dieting obsession is far from straightforward. But, ironically, it does seem that the trend has been exacerbated by food fears and society's increased focus on childhood obesity, which can leave many non-overweight youngsters stressed about their bodies.

Add to that the rise in scares about food additives and contamination, the escalating number of food allergies and intolerances and the popular, widely publicised diets of celebrities that often involve cutting out entire food groups and it is little wonder that the majority of young people now take it as given that certain people exclude certain foods most of the time. There is no easy solution, but educating children about healthy eating, that food is fuel for activity and brainpower and that wholesome fare can be enjoyed is crucial to their future relationship with food. At a young age, it is crucial that children are not overly aware of the constituents of food – calories, fat, carbohydrate and protein – as it can trigger obsessions and unhealthy eating behaviours as they grow. Our job as parents is to guide them towards a nutritious and healthy lifestyle.

GET THEM MOVING

Children are more likely to lead sedentary lifestyles than ever before. With computer games and 24-hour television at their disposal, and cars to take them to school, many fail to move around much at all. The effects can be devastating, not just to their health in later life, but to their self-esteem and sense of well-being. Active children are known to do better at school and to lead more active social lives. Here are some tips to get your children moving:

- **Buy them sporty toys** Skipping ropes, skateboards, basketball nets, pogo sticks, inline skates, baseball or cricket sets. Inject a sense of excitement with something fun and different.

➤

- **Let them play** Not every country sets specific exercise guidelines for children under the age of six, but as a guideline you could use those set by the American Academy of Pediatrics (AAP), which recommends 15 minutes a day of 'structured activity' – that is, specific games such as football, throwing a ball or swimming – for the under-fives. Aside from that, encourage plenty of 'free play': digging in a sandpit or the garden, dancing to music or playing with building bricks and toy trains all count towards activity at this age.

- **Get an hour of exercise a day** Children of school age should be getting at least an hour a day of general activity. Playground games (such as tag) and competitive sports (such as cricket, football, rounders and tennis) are ideal for developing all-round strength and cardiovascular fitness. Encourage them to cycle, swim and run as often as possible too at a rate that leaves them breathless and sweaty.

- **Be active parents** Get your kids to walk as much as possible. At the weekend drive to woodland and plan a walk of no less than 40 minutes. Take them out of their normal comfort zone. Get them to pick up the pace as often as they can. It's fine to lure them with rewards and they often enjoy it so walk to a café and promise a drink or ice cream.

- **Walk them to school** If an hour a week were spent walking instead of travelling by car, it would prevent the average person from gaining 12.7kg (2 stone/28lb) over a decade.

Start them young
— and not on ready meals

In the first year of a baby's life, the dietary angst experienced by many parents wanting to provide their children with the best nutritional springboard to life is the biggest burden of baby-dom. There is the unending pressure to breast feed and to keep it up for six months. Then there is the steaming, puréeing and freezing ice-cube blocks of sweet potato, carrot and butternut squash as a child is weaned onto solids. One false step and the fear is that your baby will at best end up a fussy eater – at worst an obesity statistic.

Commercial puréed baby products, which are effectively ready meals for babies, first soared in popularity in the 1970s when manufacturers started producing them. The global baby food industry is now worth £6 billion and is currently hurtling upmarket with baby foods based on locally produced so-called organic super-foods. Many researchers and even the nutrition advisors for UNICEF now argue that the pulp-like products are unnecessary. A growing movement suggests parents forget what is traditionally considered the first stage of weaning – purées and weaning spoons – and simply let babies feed themselves with finger food such as courgette batons, low-salt bread pieces and broccoli spears.

Consider the facts. At about six months, most babies have strong necks and can sit up if they are supported. Their hand-eye coordination has developed to the extent that they can reach out and start to grasp food and grip it in their palms. As long as they can sit up, the risk of choking on food is minimal.

Choose finger foods

Studies on 'baby-led weaning' have shown that babies introduced to finger foods and self-feeding from six months onwards
are less likely to become fussy eaters, develop allergies or refuse
foods as they get older. In many countries, a more freewheel-
ing approach is used to start babies on flavourful fare: meat is
given to babies in African countries, while the Japanese give
them fish and radishes, and the French think nothing of weaning on tomatoes and artichokes. In the West, spices are ignored
in weaning guidelines and parents advised not to introduce
them to the diet until children are toddlers – yet the only evidence against including them seems to be cultural rather than
scientific.

The argument is all the more convincing when you consider
that many top-selling baby foods lack vital nutrients essential
for growth and protection against illness. Researchers at the
University of Greenwich in the UK found that many of the most
popular brands contain less than a fifth of the recommended
daily supply of calcium, magnesium, zinc, iron and other crucial minerals. Infants of six months plus given one ready-made
meat jar and one vegetable jar on top of 600ml (20fl oz/1 pint)
of formula milk would not be getting enough calcium, essential
for building strong bones and teeth, regulating the heart beat
and ensuring that the blood clots properly. Also lacking would
be magnesium, which is important for bone health, and copper
and selenium which boost the immune system.

Foods to avoid

Of course, there are certain foods that are more risky to your baby
because of their texture or shape – nuts, for instance, may cause
choking – and obviously unhealthy additions to a baby's diet such

as salt, sugar, additives, raw honey, cow's milk and sweetened or fizzy drinks should be avoided. But feeding your baby real food from the outset in a move towards baby-led weaning makes an appealing choice in every way. A great starting point for researching this area is the website babyledweaning.com.

Breakfast cereals

As risible as the idea of having a 'dessert for breakfast' may sound, that could be what you are giving your children every morning. Many breakfast cereals aimed at children are so full of sugar that consumers groups such as Which? suggest two-thirds of them should be placed in the biscuit and confectionary aisles of supermarkets. In effect, they are no better for your children than, say, a chocolate brownie or a slice of Victoria sponge for breakfast.

In the recommended 40g (1½oz) serving (although many of us pour far more than that into a bowl), there is often the equivalent of 3½ teaspoons of sugar. Add the average serving of 125ml (4fl oz) of semi-skimmed milk, with its own intrinsic sugars, and it totals over 5 teaspoons of sugar that you are feeding your children before school. Some brands have as many as 8 teaspoons of sugar per bowl; 35 per cent of the weight of a children's cereal packet can be sugar. But how can we tell the wholesome breakfast wheat from the sugary chaff?

Added vitamins do not necessarily mean 'healthy'

It's not always straightforward. A lack of consistent labelling across brands makes it difficult for families to identify the healthier options quickly. And misleading suggestions about cereals being vitamin-packed health foods can lure us into thinking that a sugary cereal is a virtuous choice. Clever marketing by manufacturers has helped to convince parents that sugary cereals are fun, benign, and something all children should eat. Using words such as 'honey' to describe a highly sweetened product gives the impression that it is a better choice than a sugar-laden cereal. This is simply not the case. In a packet of honey loops cereal, for example, after oats, wheat and barley the most prevalent ingredients are sugar, honey and glucose syrup – basically, all forms of sugar – which explains why it comprises 34 per cent sugar.

The salt problem

It's not just sugar levels that are problematic. Since manufacturers were taken to task about the high salt levels in children's cereals a few years ago, many have reformulated their products to meet acceptable targets. Nevertheless, 16 per cent of breakfast cereals tested by Which? in 2012, including Nestlé cheerios and Kellogg's rice krispies, were found to contain unacceptably high levels of salt.

Fortifying foods is only part of the picture

Manufacturers make much of the fact that many breakfast cereals are fortified with vitamins and that they contribute valuable nutrients to children's diets. Of the best-selling brands, many contain added thiamin, riboflavin, niacin, vitamin B_6, folic acid, vitamin B_{12}, iron and calcium. In response to concerns about the rise in rickets among children – 82 per cent of paediatric dieticians have reported a rise in the disease in recent years

– some manufacturers have started adding vitamin D to cereals. The supplementation with synthetically produced vitamins and minerals via breakfast cereals might be considered laudable, but my concern is that it doesn't address the root of the problem.

The rise in rickets is due to the fact that children spend time indoors watching television and playing computer games and, even when they do play outside, are often smothered head to toe in sunblock or sunscreen, meaning that their exposure to the sun – the main provider of vitamin D – is vastly reduced. Scientists have linked the causes of rickets, which is character-ised by weak bones and bowed legs, to a lack of vitamin D. In the long term, a deficiency of the vitamin can lead to illnesses including cancer, heart disease, high blood pressure and mul-tiple sclerosis. There is no doubt that children need vitamin D, and other vitamins and minerals, in their diet, but I am deeply sceptical about whether providing it in a bowl of sugary break-fast cereal is the best solution in the long term when the vita-min is readily available in natural sources – both from the great outdoors and from fresh foods in our diet.

For all the gloom, there are wise breakfast choices that will set your child up for a healthy start. When you are buying break-fast products, look out for salt and sugar contents rather than focusing solely on calories and fat, because children need these to grow.

Healthier breakfast choices

Porridge (per 50g (1¾oz) serving: calories 178; fat 4.0g; sugars 0.5g; salt trace). Plain porridge oats are known to have a low glycaemic index, which means that they provide a long-lasting energy boost – perfect to sustain energy levels through to lunch time. If made with milk, nearly all of the sugars are natural milk lactose; if made with water, porridge contains only 0.4g of sugars per serving. Oats provide about half the GDA of healthy beta-glucan soluble fibre. What's more, in a study published in the *Economic Journal* children who were in the habit of eating porridge for breakfast before their third birthday had improved scores in reading and problem-solving tests compared with their peers. But it's never too late to change.

Weetabix (per 37.5g serving, 2 biscuits: calories 134; fat 0.8g; sugars 1.7g; salt 0.24g). Original weetabix biscuits are made from 95 per cent wholegrain wheat and relatively little added sugar – it provides only 4 per cent of the total weight of each biscuit. Although they are fortified with a range of vitamins, you will enhance your kids' intake by topping the cereal with fresh fruit.

Crisped rice (per 50g (1¾oz) serving before milk is added: calories 191; fat 0.5g; sugar 5g; salt 0.5g). Although not the best breakfast choice because, like most commercial cereals, they are highly processed, crisped rice cereals are lower in sugar than many options and a far better choice than their chocolate-containing or sugar-coated counterparts. Beware, though, some brands have even higher levels of salt – up to 0.9g per serving – and there is little fibre, so add fresh or dried fruit to boost it.

Boiled egg (calories 80; fat 5.8g; sugars trace; salt trace). For a sugar- and additive-free start to the day, there is little better than a boiled egg. Naturally packed with vitamins and minerals the protein content will keep kids stoked up until lunchtime, particularly if you add some toasted wholemeal bread soldiers for added fibre.

MORE HEALTHY (AND CONVENIENT) IDEAS

- A slice of wholemeal toast and fruit.

- Plain yoghurt topped with fresh fruit and a sprinkle of muesli.

- Eggy bread (bread dipped in beaten egg and fried) with ham or grilled bacon.

- Wholemeal pancakes filled with fromage frais and fruit.

- Bircher muesli: many children find regular muesli too 'chewy'. So, instead, try Swiss Bircher muesli which is softened by soaking the oats in fruit juice or milk overnight. Add grated apple and some dried fruit in the morning for a wholesome and delicious treat.

Lunchboxes

In the UK, half of all children now take a packed lunch to school. Concerns about the quality of school meals has seen the number of children taking a lunch with them rise steadily in recent years. But is it always a healthy move to make their lunch at home? Research published in the *Journal of Epidemiology and Community Health* by researchers at the University of Leeds in the UK revealed that a paltry 1 per cent of typical lunchbox contents meet government nutritional standards for school meals. The findings were described as 'appalling' by children's health campaigners, who want all children to be given free, nutritious school meals.

In the same study, about 82 per cent of lunchboxes were revealed to contain foods high in fat, salt and sugar, with more than seven out of ten containing crisps, and 60 per cent containing a chocolate bar or a biscuit. Only one in five packed lunches analysed by the Leeds researchers contained any vegetables or salad, and only about half included a piece of fruit. Overall, most failed to meet the necessary levels of vitamin A, folate, iron and zinc; fruit was the food least likely to be eaten when provided in a lunchbox, whereas confectionery was most likely to be eaten when provided.

Given the contents of the average UK lunchbox, it is not surprising that children are consuming double their daily recommended maximum of sugar, half the suggested salt intake plus high levels of saturated fat in their midday school meal.

Beware of snacks aimed at children

What is even more shocking is that if you buy popular lunchbox items and snack foods marketed at children, many of which are billed as healthy, your child's lunchbox could easily contain 60g of sugar, the equivalent of 12 teaspoons, making the meal as sugary as 10 McDonald's sugar donuts or nearly a pint of Coca-Cola. None of us would purposely feed those levels to our children, and so good choices are crucial. By far the best foods are fresh and natural produce such as fruit, vegetable crudités, unsweetened yoghurts, dark chocolate and chunks of cheese.

Take extra care when it comes to choosing ready-made lunch-box products targeted at children, as they can be among the worst offenders on the supermarket shelves. Take the Dairylea lunchables range. Its ham and cheese crackers sound straightforward enough, but they contain two-thirds of a 5-year-olds daily maximum salt intake and 2.8g of sugar. The ham used contains only 85 per cent meat and the cheese filling only 73 per cent cheese. The rest is made up with flavourings, stabilisers and other ingredients that are highly unnecessary in a child's lunchbox. Or Fruit Factory fruit strings, often positioned in the dried fruit section, which the manufacturers claim to be 'bursting with fruit juice concentrate' – not exactly something to shout about, as it is reconstituted with water. They are also bursting with 50 per cent sugar, containing no fewer than three different types – glucose syrup, sugar and fructose syrup – and are no better than a bag of jelly babies.

A seemingly healthy cereal bar can also be a sugary nightmare. Take Kellogg's frosties cereal bar: it provides your growing child with no less than five different types of sugar: sweetened condensed milk, HFCS, sugar, invert sugar syrup and fructose.

Ideas for lunchboxes

An excellent reference point for school lunch ideas is the website of the School Food Trust (schoolfoodtrust.org.uk) where you will find low-cost and low-effort lunchbox-meal ideas for children. Here are some of the top choices:

Cheddar cheese sticks or cubes Pre-packed sticks of mild Cheddar cheese are great if your child likes the idea of opening something, but you could also send them with a slice or cube of cheese – cheaper and just as tasty. Add a few cream crackers (or bread) and a slice of ham.

Bottle of water Getting children to drink water in place of sugary drinks is a hugely positive step. Researchers at the Institute of Psychiatry found that teenagers' brains work less efficiently when they become dehydrated, making tasks such as problem solving far harder. Hot conditions, such as poorly ventilated classrooms or exam halls, could lead to pupils becoming dehydrated enough to affect the neural activity in key parts of their brains which, as a result, have to work harder to achieve the same tasks. The effects of all that exam revision could be enhanced if they take a drink of water into the exam hall. Pupils who sipped water during an exam did up to 10 per cent better than those who did not – the difference between a grade.

Raisins (calories 125; fat 0g; sugar 31.0g; salt 0g). Raisins are naturally high in sugar, but contain no added sweeteners. They are a good source of potassium, which is important in regulating blood pressure. They are also a significant source of the antioxidants that help fight disease. Dried fruit should not be eaten in excess, so no more than 25g (1oz) a day for young children is best, and it makes a much better snack than jelly sweets.

Miniature bar of milk or dark chocolate A daily bar of milk chocolate in a children's lunchbox is not advisable because of its relatively high sugar and fat content, but as an occasional treat the mini chocolate bar is fine. Milk chocolate contains 15g of sugar so dark chocolate is a healthier option.

Slice of malt loaf Since it is packed with dried fruit, malt loaf is a good source of iron and potassium as well as fibre. A far better lunchbox treat than biscuits and other highly refined, pre-made cakes.

Home-made flapjacks with seeds and nuts Commercial flapjacks tend to be loaded with sugar and HFCS as well as other unnecessary ingredients. Make your own with oats, brown sugar and butter and add flavour accordingly – desiccated coconut, nuts, seeds and dried fruits – for a healthier treat.

Plain popcorn A worthy treat (see page 190), just make sure it's not smothered in sugar or toffee.

Organic yoghurt If you are going to send your child to school with a yoghurt in their lunchbox, make sure it doesn't contain thickeners such as guar gum and rice starch along with lots of added sugars (see below). What's more, many children's yoghurt and fromage frais products are promoted as being 'without fruit bits', but it's not a great idea to allow children to get accustomed to eating smooth foods. A variety of textures and tastes is crucial to the development of their taste buds. Check that the yoghurt you buy has no added sugar and that it is sweetened instead with fruit purée or concentrated apple juice, or flavour your own as suggested below.

THE CHILDREN'S YOGHURT CONUNDRUM

Let's make it clear: yoghurt is good for children. It provides calcium for their growing bones and it has been shown to reduce a child's risk of developing tooth decay. In a study from the University of Tokyo, children who ate yoghurt at least four times a week had reduced the chances of developing cavities by 22 per cent once they reached the age of three compared to those who ate it less than once a week.

When researchers and specialists talk about the benefits of yoghurt, however, they are, by and large, not talking about children's yoghurts. Yoghurts aimed at the children's market can be loaded with far too much sugar or, worse, are bought topped with chocolate chips or psychedelic sugar sprinkles. Parents are pestered to buy them because there is a popular cartoon character on the pack, but it's what's inside that matters.

▶

Home-made fruit yoghurt

In general, plain yoghurt to which you add fruit, some compote or purée is best. That way you can control how much sugar (if any) is added. Adding a teaspoon of honey is no bad move considering some children's yoghurts contain the equivalent of 5–6 teaspoons per pot, although fruit alone should supply sufficient sweetness.

As always, be careful not to swallow all the claims on packaging. One popular yoghurt brand was banned from showing an advert that claimed it supported children's natural defences against disease. The Advertising Standards Authority in the UK ruled that the claims that it could help protect school-age youngsters against illness were not supported by any evidence. It's an all too familiar story.

Know your juices

How do you tell which juice is the best buy for your child? Below is a guide to what the confusing terms on juice bottles really mean. In general, it is best for children to drink milk or water to stay hydrated. In terms of juice, make sure it is unsweetened either with sugar or artificial sweeteners. Too much fruit juice or too many smoothies can play havoc with young teeth and also waistlines, so limit to one a day (see page 266). It is a good idea to water juice down in the way you would use orange squash.

100 per cent freshly squeezed juice This is usually prepared with the pith and pulp of the squeezed or pressed fruit and needs to be drunk quickly. Even the freshest 'freshly pressed or squeezed' juice has often been prepared more than a day before-hand, so it is best to make your own. The amount of vitamin C in a carton of orange juice deteriorates by 2 per cent per day after opening.

Unsweetened fruit juice Despite the label, this can contain up to 15g (½oz) of natural sugars found in the fruit per 1 litre (1¾ pints). This is because when fruits are juiced only the sugars remain, because all the fibre has been removed, so fruit juice is a concentrated form of sugars.

Sweetened fruit juice contains up to 100g (3½oz) of sugar per 1 litre (1¾ pints). It is pasteurised, which can destroy important vitamins contained in the fruit.

Long-life juice is pasteurised to extend its shelf life and contains only half the vitamin C of fresh juice. Folate levels are also affected by processing and storing. It is often sweetened.

From concentrates The juice goes through a process where all the water is removed – and with it much of the flavour. Sugar is sometimes added. It is then re-mixed with water when required.

Not-from-concentrate juice Often the liquid is pasteurised and 'de-aerated' so that it doesn't oxidise. It's then put into huge storage tanks where it can be kept for up to one year. Chemical flavours are often added before the drinks are packaged.

Fruit drink These need contain only 5 per cent juice, although some contain more. They are also likely to be highly sweetened.

Fruit flavour drink These contain no fruit or juice. They can be artificially flavoured to taste like fruit.

CHAPTER ELEVEN

Eating out

FOR MANY OF US, EATING OUT is now a way of life rather than an occasional treat. On average, people in the UK will consume a staggering 2,453 takeaway meals – that's about 46 a year – by the time they are 62. Surveys suggest this amount is reached by gobbling away 188 kebabs, 322 Chinese dishes, 368 pizzas, 375 burgers, 312 portions of fish and chips and 92 hot dogs in a lifetime. That's not to mention the meals eaten out in restaurants and cafés, something that has become an increasingly common practice in many people's lifestyles.

When it comes to losing weight, part of the problem with this habit is that we have little control over how restaurant and takeaway food is cooked or of the portion sizes we will be given. Generally, foods eaten outside the home are higher in fat, and studies show that people who regularly eat out have higher intakes of fat, salt and calories overall. Surprisingly, though, it is not the much-maligned fast-food chains like McDonald's and Burger King that are always the worst culprits.

Healthier-sounding and more upmarket restaurants, such as gourmet burger outlets, organic pizza companies and noodle bars, contribute as significantly to our fat and calorie consumption outside the home.

Since there is no legal requirement for restaurants to provide nutritional and calorie information (although many now do – see page 231), it is often impossible to tell what you are eating. Even some restaurants that do post calorie counts have been found to do so inaccurately. A survey by nutritionists at Tufts University in Boston, USA, found 'substantial inaccuracy' for the amounts of calories listed on menus. Indeed, they suggested that nearly 20 per cent of dishes are packed with up to 1,000 more calories than are listed. At one chain, a bowl of chicken and gnocchi soup was listed as containing 529 calories on the menu. When the scientists analysed its ingredients they found it contained 246 more than that per portion. Of course, we have no way of telling if the information we are being fed is accurate, so my advice is to consider it a loose guideline and not to take everything as gospel.

Reading between the lines at restaurants

Often what's omitted from nutritional information is as important as what's provided. High salt and fat contents as well as hidden ingredients are commonplace. Pizzas in restaurants and from takeaway chains have been shown to be twice as salty as those bought from a supermarket. And a local government survey of Indian and Chinese restaurants in England and Wales found high levels of salt and saturated fat in meals at 223 takeaways, while 20 per cent of supposedly nut-free chicken tikka meals did, in fact, contain nuts when they were tested.

Worse, the government researchers found one-fifth of chicken tikka masala and pilau rice meals contained illegally high levels of colourings, including sunset yellow (E110), allura red (E129), tartrazine (E102) and ponceau 4R (E124). The government has called for a voluntary ban on these additives due to a reported link with hyperactivity in children. An analysis of 11 sweet-and-sour chicken meals from Chinese takeaways revealed that one contained levels of the colourings above the permitted maximum of 500mg per 1kg (2lb 4oz).

Choose well and, of course, you can eat out without busting the calorie and fat bank. What matters is selecting wisely off the menu and knowing the pitfalls to avoid. If you know you are going to be eating out or having a takeaway meal, plan ahead so that you eat sensibly for the rest of the day, keeping calorie, fat and sugar levels under healthy control.

WATER MIGHT HELP YOU LOSE WEIGHT

Slimmers can lose an average of 2.25kg (5lb) extra if they drink two glasses of water three times a day before meals, according to one study published in the *Journal of Obesity*. Two groups of adults followed the same low-calorie diet, one group drinking water before meals. After 12 weeks, those drinking water lost about 7.03kg (15.5lb) whereas the others lost about 5kg (11lb). The theory is that water fills up the stomach, so you feel more full when you eat your meal.

What menus can tell us

In some places, such as New York City, California, Seattle and Massachusetts, authorities have made it a legal requirement for the majority of restaurants to provide calorie information on their menus. Both the Australian and the UK governments also encourage all food outlets to provide details of precisely how many calories are in their meals, and you will now find such information everywhere, from fish and chip shops to Michelin-starred restaurants and at chains such as Pizza Hut, KFC, Burger King and Pret a Manger.

Do we really want – or need – to know? A survey of 1,000 people who ate at the Real Greek chain of restaurants in the UK revealed that many had an inaccurate perception of the calories in everyday foods. Almost 70 per cent of people thought, for instance, that a fillet steak (210 calories) was more fattening than a cheese sandwich (260) and 45 per cent of people thought an apple (79 calories) contained more calories than a bowl of rice (up to 400).

In New York, surveys have shown that people eat 50–100 fewer calories per meal when eating out since the labelling rules were brought into force. It might not seem a lot, but when you consider that eating an extra 20 calories a day can result in 900g (2lb) of weight gained in a year, it can make a difference.

Drink a glass of orange juice with your fast food meal

Researchers at the University of Buffalo found that the flavonoid substances in orange juice help to neutralise the oxidative and inflammatory stress generated by fast food like burgers, pizzas and chips. In turn, they suggest, that could also prevent blood vessel damage. Two particular flavonoids in the juice, naringenin and hesperidin, which are major antioxidants, had a potent effect on preventing inflammation, something that did not happen when participants drank water or a sugary drink with the meal. What it won't do is aid weight loss, though. So be careful not to add juice to your meal too often.

Eating with friends

People we dine with can have a powerful influence on how much we eat. Through studying our behaviour patterns, psychologists know that we adjust our food intake – up or down – to match that of our fellow diners and that we tend to eat more with others than when dining alone. When Dutch researchers invited 70 pairs of women to dine together in a laboratory that was set up to look like a restaurant they found the women, who didn't know each other, tended to take bites of food at roughly the same time and mimic each other's overall eating behaviour. This mirroring effect was three times more common at the beginning of the meal than at the end, suggesting that the subjects were trying to impress each other and were eating more to be socially accepted by their peers and not just because they were hungry.

Eating with friends and people we know, such as work colleagues, can also mean that we pack away more calories, as demonstrated in another study, published in the *American Journal of Clinical Nutrition*, in which researchers found that 9 to 15-year-olds, regardless of their weight, tended to eat more when they had the chance to snack with a friend than when they were with a peer they did not know. But the biggest calorie intakes were seen when an overweight child snacked with an overweight friend. The message? Be careful what you eat and who you eat it with.

Don't eat a takeaway in front of the TV

Having your meal on your lap leads to 'mindless eating' and the consumption of a third more calories than you would normally eat. What's shown in commercial breaks can make matters worse. A study at Yale University in the US showed that adults who watched TV ads for unhealthy foods ate much more than those who saw ads that featured messages about good nutrition or healthy food. Another test found that 45 per cent more snack food was eaten if food commercials were shown during a programme.

TOP SWAP TIP

When eating out:

- Pass on the breadsticks, garlic bread and bread basket, to save 100–400 calories.

- Have soup as a starter. Studies have shown you will consume 20 per cent fewer calories in your overall meal if you do.

- Fill up on side orders of salad and green or red vegetables, not extra potatoes and pasta.

- Choose a starter or entrée-sized portion as a main course. Often you can cut calories and fat by at least one-third.

- Opt for food that is grilled, baked, steamed or poached when you can. Avoid deep-fried dishes or those swimming in creamy sauces.

Pizzas

In their original and most basic form in Italy, pizzas are a truly balanced meal: a thin bread base; a fresh tomato and herb sauce topping, packed with antioxidants and beneficial substances such as lycopene (which is present in tomatoes in greater amounts when they are cooked); and a little cheese, which gives you calcium and protein. Add a green salad and you have additional fibre with a host of immune-boosting nutrients. Perfect.

Pizza restaurants and chains claim to use this basic recipe, but they also add their own spin on things – and the result isn't always a pretty picture. Surveys by the medical lobbying group in the UK, Consensus Action on Salt and Health, revealed that takeaway and restaurant pizzas can be as salty as those that are sold in supermarkets which have already been found to be overly salty. Half of all the pizzas tested contained the entire maximum daily recommended amount of salt for an adult: 6.0g. One particular pepperoni pizza contained a whopping 10.7g or 2.73 per cent salt, making it saltier than the Atlantic Ocean where the seawater is 2.5 per cent salt.

UK government targets are to reduce salt content in pizzas to a maximum of 1.25g per 100g (3½oz) by 2013. At present, only 16 per cent of takeaway pizzas meet this guideline. In the meantime, make wise choices where you can. Some chains (such as Pizza Express) give only calorie counts and don't provide information on salt, sugars and fats, which can mean that decision making is more difficult. Others (such as Pizza Hut and Zizzis) provide detailed information, meaning that the decision-making process is that much more straightforward.

SWAP ▸ Dough sticks with garlic aioli

Per portion: calories 624; fat 57.1g; sugars 13.1g; salt 1.25g

Dough sticks are generally brushed with olive oil and rosemary and served with aioli – a garlic and oil dip. You could eat a main pasta dish for fewer calories than this as a starter. Drop the aioli and you lose much of the fat and 222 calories – better still, choose something else.

FOR ▸ Bruschetta with goat's cheese and tomatoes

Per portion: calories 329; fat 27.6g; sugar 6.8g; salt 0.25g

Bread brushed with olive oil and topped with goat's cheese, plum tomatoes and roasted peppers with a balsamic dressing. It's best to avoid starters, but it does save you 295 calories over the dough sticks.

DID YOU KNOW?

Beware garlic bread with cheese on the pizza menu. This fat-laden version of already fatty garlic bread is a favourite in pizza chains. The dough is made with bread and oil; cheese is then added to the mix, so there's little wonder that it is higher in fat and calories. A plain cheese and tomato pizza would contain less.

SWAP ▸ Pepperoni stuffed-crust pizza

Per portion: calories 1,300; fat 55g; sugar 12.3g; salt 4.92g

An average 28cm (11in) pizza (a large version would contain 2,368 calories) has a cheese-stuffed crust and is loaded with lots of high-fat, low-nutrient pepperoni. With 55g of fat and almost 5g of salt (the daily maximum is 6g), this should be off anyone's wish list.

FOR ▸ Regular vegetarian pizza

Per portion: calories 894; fat 28.8g; sugar 12.5g; salt 3.42g

Choose a thinner, 'Italian' base over a stuffed crust and you automatically have less fat than the dreaded deep-pan or stuffed-crust variety. In addition, you can opt for a pizza topped with spinach, cherry tomatoes, peppers, red onions and mushrooms offering far more nutrients than pepperoni. It saves you 354 calories, but is still very high in salt.

––––––

SWAP ▸ Regular quattro stagioni pizza

Per portion: calories 1,320; fat 76g; sugar 10.7g; salt 9g

This unassuming classic pizza may have its good points – mushrooms, tomatoes and artichokes – but they are far outweighed by the bad ones. Ham, pepperoni and cheese mean that it provides almost 75 per cent of a woman's recommended daily calorie intake (2,000) and over half of a man's (2,500) as well as very high fat levels and 150 per cent of daily salt intakes – in one sitting. A nutritional horror.

FOR ▸ Regular mushroom pizza

Per portion: calories 791; fat 25.1g; sugar 8g; salt 4.5g

A much safer choice. Here you get a topping of field mushrooms, mozzarella and thyme. Add a green salad for a little more vitamin C. This pizza is still very high in salt, but it has 521 fewer calories.

TOP SWAP TIP

Here's what to avoid and what to choose when eating at the pizzeria:

- Avoid stuffed crusts and deep-pan bases. They are loaded with extra fat and calories. The thinner the base the better in terms of calories.

- Choose vegetable toppings over meat and extra cheese toppings. If you do want meat, opt for ham and pineapple as opposed to the 'meaty feast' variety. All pizzas contain some cheese for protein unless specified. Just don't add extra.

- Seafood and vegetarian options often contain the least calories so are worth checking out.

- Steer clear of starters such as garlic bread, bruschetta, dough sticks and dough balls served with garlic butter. A typical starter of 4 slices of garlic bread contains 376 calories and 17.7g of fat.

- Share a pizza. Halve it and fill the other half of your plate with a green salad and you will have cut down on calories considerably. Some pizzerias now offer 'lighter' pizzas which are half salad, half pizza.

SWAP ▶ Meat and veg-topped pizza

Per portion: calories 1,928; fat 72.8g; sugars 34.4g; salt 10.4g

Topped with sausage, ham, pepperoni and ground beef as well as more favourable pineapple, green pepper, mushrooms, onion and sweetcorn, this pizza can have almost the total daily amount of calories for a woman (2,000) in all of its eight slices. Its fat and salt levels are colossal, with more than 1.5 times the amount of salt we should get in a day (even if you do share it with someone it contains almost all of your daily salt).

FOR ▸ Regular ham and pineapple

Per portion: calories 602; fat 15.8g; sugars 11.3g; salt 3g

This four-slice pizza should be more than enough for an adult. If you must have meat, ham and pineapple is a reasonable choice in terms of fat. This contains less than one-third of the calories of the meat and veg-topped pizza. It is still high in salt, though, containing half the daily maximum.

ADD UP THE EXTRAS

It's not just pizzas that are calorie laden. The extras you are offered in a pizzeria can also head straight for the waistline. Check out the calorie content of these popular side orders (per average portion):

Coleslaw: 268 calories

Potato wedges: 380 calories

Barbecued chicken wings: 353 calories

Bacon bits: 100 calories

Croutons: 94 calories

Blue cheese dressing: 64 calories

Caesar dressing: 46 calories

Reduced-fat thousand island dressing: 47 calories

▶

Potato salad: 98 calories

Mixed olives: 131 calories

Calamari: 439 calories

Antipasto: 383 calories

Grated Parmesan (added at the table): 20 calories

Chilli oil (added at the table): 108 calories

Indian meals

For many people in the UK Indian food has become a long-standing favourite; it accounts for two-thirds of all meals eaten out. Indeed, one of the UK's top takeaway meals is chicken tikka masala served with pilau rice. In terms of finding which dishes are healthy choices, and which are not, however, Indian restaurants can be a minefield.

There are many positive aspects of Indian cuisine. Traditionally, south Asian diets contain a huge variety of vegetables as well as dishes that are rich in whole grains and pulses, including lentils, peas and dried beans such as kidney beans, chickpeas and black-eyed beans. Tandoori dishes contain very little sauce and, because the food is baked instead of fried, it is generally much lower in fat and calories than many curries. Turmeric, the bright yellow spice used in many curry dishes, is thought to have numerous healing properties. One study discovered that a compound found in turmeric, called curcumin, may help to fight and prevent a common yet very serious kind of fatty liver disease called non-alcoholic steatohepatitis. The disease can be a result of obesity and weight gain, and it affects 3–4 per cent of adults.

Beware the fatty choices

You can unwittingly end up with dishes that contain a lot of cream, oil and fat. Indeed, one survey found that the average Indian takeaway has 23.2g of saturated fat, 3.2g more than a woman should eat in a day. The UK's favourite dish, chicken tikka masala and pilau rice, includes, on average, 116 per cent of a person's GDA of fat as well as 92 per cent of their salt allowance.

WHAT IS GHEE?

Ghee, a clarified butter, is widely used in Indian cooking and is partly responsible for the high fat content of many dishes. Prepared from cow or buffalo milk, it is clarified by removing most of the water and milk solids so that all that is left is pure fat. It gets a bad name because it consists of approximately 65 per cent saturated animal fats, previously thought to raise cholesterol. But the saturated fat it contains is mostly the easily digested form of short-chain fatty acids that might actually help to strengthen and develop cell membranes whereas long-chain acids increase the risks of blood clots and cancer. It also contains 3 per cent linoleic acid, a source of antioxidants that protect the body against free radicals and help to prevent serious health diseases. Several studies, including one published in the *Journal of Nutrition Biochemistry*, suggest that rather than raising cholesterol levels in the body as was previously thought, ghee can actually help to lower them by improving the ratio of high-density lipoprotein, HDL or 'good cholesterol', to low-density lipoprotein, LDL or 'bad cholesterol'. But ghee

▶

is still a fat so shouldn't be over-used, as too much of any kind of fat in the diet leads to weight gain. A low-fat version of ghee, developed in India, that claims to have 80–85 per cent less saturated fat compared to normal ghee is now available.

SWAP ▸ Meat samosa

Per portion: calories 320; fat 14.6g; sugar 3.4g; salt 0.9g

Samosas are deep-fried parcels of meat or vegetables which, naturally, means they contain a lot of fat. If you have one samosa and one onion bhaji (250 calories for the bhaji) you will consume more than one-quarter of the daily calories for a woman.

FOR ▸ 2 poppadums with lime pickle

Per portion: calories 200; fat 5.9g; sugar 2.9g; salt 1.1g

Poppadums are made with lentil flour and vegetable oil. At 65 calories each, they are a relatively good starter. Lime pickle has 70 calories per tablespoon, so all in all, this swap saves you 120 calories and almost 9g of fat.

––––––––––

SWAP ▸ Chicken korma

Per portion: calories 820; fat 42.4g; sugar 12.8g; salt 2.2g

Coconut milk and almonds give this dish its distinctive creamy taste. They also mean it is among the highest in fat and calories of all Indian dishes. Add pilau rice and you are looking at 1,470 calories: three-quarters of the daily amount for a woman.

FOR ▸ Chicken jalfrezi

Per portion: calories 420; fat 18g; sugar 4.0g; salt 2.4g

A jalfrezi is made by marinating meat and then frying it in spices to produce a dry, thick sauce. Peppers and onions are added plus chillies to produce varying levels of heat. It's a much better choice than korma and it saves you almost half the calories.

––––––––––

SWAP ▸ Peshwari naan

Per portion: calories 310; fat 9.3g; sugar 7.7g; salt 0.7g

A sweet-tasting bread filled with sultanas, coconut and honey peshwari naan adds considerably to the fat and calorie content of your meal when served as a side order.

FOR ▸ Plain naan

Per portion: calories 275; fat 5.8g; sugar 2.8g; salt 0.8g

A better choice than peshwari, a plain naan will save you 35 calories. You could go even lower with a chapatti, which contains only 120 calories per portion.

––––––––––

SWAP ▸ Chicken tikka masala

Per portion: calories 680; fat 40.4g; sugar 21.2g; salt 4.6g

This most popular Indian dish also happens to be loaded with calories and fat. Add a naan bread and rice and you have almost 1,500 calories. Chicken tikka masala also contains almost 75 per cent of the daily salt intake.

FOR ▶ Chicken vindaloo

Per portion: calories 552; fat 29.4g; sugar 18.9g; salt 3.2g

A hot curry (which sometimes means you eat less of it), a vindaloo is seasoned with red chillies, tamarind and other spices, such as ginger, cumin and mustard seeds. It saves you 128 calories per serving and halves your fat intake. It is still high in fat and salt, but is a better choice.

———

SWAP ▶ Beef keema

Per portion: calories 780; fat 28.6g; sugars 19g; salt 3.1g

A beef keema is made from minced meat that is stewed or fried and combined with peas or potatoes, onions, garlic and ginger. It is often used as the filling for meat samosas but is relatively high in calories and fat. It also contains one-third of the daily maximum for salt.

FOR ▶ Tandoori chicken

Per portion: calories 305; fat 16.3g; sugars 14.3g; salt 2g

This is among the best choices on an Indian restaurant menu and contains less fat than many dishes. The Indian version of roast chicken, a tandoori is cooked with yoghurt and spices in a tandoor (clay oven). A great swap that saves you 460 calories.

———

TOP SWAP TIP

Here's what to avoid and what to choose when eating out at an Indian restaurant:

- Avoid creamy curries like korma, masala (containing ground almonds and cream) and pasanda (cooked in cream) because these are higher in fat. Choose tomato-based sauces like bhuna, rhogan and jalfrezi.

- Steer clear of deep-fried starters, such as onion bhaji and meat or vegetable samosas. If anything, opt for a poppadum, which are 65 calories each.

- Vegetable, chicken and prawn curries tend to be lower in fat, and sometimes calories, than those containing lamb or beef.

- Choose boiled rice (370 calories per portion) rather than pilau rice (650 calories per portion) because pilau is made with added oil.

- The best dips are the cucumber-based raita and tomato sambal (chopped tomato and onion) each containing about 20 calories per tablespoon. Avoid mango chutney, because it has 70 calories per tablespoon.

Chinese

In the popularity stakes, Chinese and Far Eastern cuisines have usurped Indian for the top spot. Yet, as much as we love it, Chinese food has a poor reputation when it comes to healthy choices. With rice-heavy meals and fatty meat dishes that are

often seasoned with the heavily criticised monosodium glutamate (MSG, see below), the general consensus is that if you eat
too much it will cause weight gain and heart disease.

WHAT IS MSG?

Invented by a chemist over a century ago, monosodium
glutamate (MSG) is a salt of glutamic acid, which is an
amino acid and building block of protein. MSG is made by
fermenting molasses or wheat. It has no smell or flavour
of its own but is used to bring out the savoury taste of
processed foods, sauces and instant meals. It is also widely
used by some (but not all) Chinese restaurants. About
50 years ago, a report in the *New England Journal of
Medicine* suggested MSG was responsible for so-called
Chinese restaurant syndrome – a complaint that caused
numbness in the neck, general weakness and palpitations
– although the evidence was never substantiated. People
have complained that MSG seasoning has caused asthma
attacks, heart conditions and depression, although no link
with these conditions has been scientifically confirmed.
Studies do suggest that there is a link with obesity, however. In one study, conducted at the University of North
Carolina, it was found that people who use MSG as a flavour enhancer in their food are more likely to be overweight
or obese, compared with others with similar lifestyles who
do not use it, even though they have the same amount
of physical activity and total calorie intake. Again, many
experts dispute such findings. What's certain is that MSG
is an unnecessary flavour enhancer and we can enjoy our
Chinese meals perfectly well without it.

As with Indian food, there can also be hidden, unwanted extras if you opt for Chinese food when you eat out or order a take-away. In a government analysis of sweet-and-sour chicken and fried rice from 133 Chinese restaurants in England and Wales, it was found that the dish contained 119 per cent of the recommended salt intake and 16 teaspoons of sugar, 75 per cent of the daily limit. On many occasions, the meat used in sweet-and-sour *chicken* dishes was actually turkey. And a survey by the consumers association Which? revealed that the average Chinese takeaway meal contains 1,436 calories, 4.7g of salt (nearly 75 per cent of the daily amount) and 60.4g of fat, only slightly less than the limit for an adult woman in a day – 70g.

There are many foods on the Chinese menu that don't fall into these categories, however. Navigating the maze of which are fattening and which aren't can be tricky, but among the best swaps are the following:

SWAP ▶ Sweet–and–sour chicken

Per portion: calories 670; fat 32.5g; sugar 19.3g; salt 3.7g

Sweet-and-sour chicken is among the worst dishes for fat and calories on the Chinese menu. It consists of deep-fried chicken pieces in a tangy sauce, and it contains almost half the calories a woman needs in a day and over half her limit of salt. And that's before you add rice.

FOR ▶ Chinese chicken curry

Per portion: calories 430; fat 20g; sugar 17.5g; salt 4g

A much better option if you are looking for a chicken dish, although a Chinese chicken curry still contains quite high levels of fat and a very high salt content. This is a once-in-a-while dish, not a regular choice. Still, you save 240 calories over the sweet-and-sour dish.

SWAP ▶ Crispy duck and 4 pancakes

Per portion: calories 800; fat 29g; sugar 33g; salt 4.1g

You won't get a nutritional profile much worse than this at a Chinese restaurant. The fat and calories come from the duck, which is served in its skin. Duck is a fatty bird and most of the fat is found just beneath the skin. If you want to eat crispy duck, eat a smaller portion of the duck and sauce, and add more cucumber and onions to lessen the calories. But it's really best avoided.

FOR ▶ Beef and black bean sauce

Per portion: calories 460; fat 22.2g; sugar 7.5g; salt 2.8g

A reasonable choice in terms of fat and sugar. The beans add more protein and the green peppers add vitamin C. You save almost half the calories compared with the crispy duck and pancakes.

TOP SWAP TIP

Here's what to avoid and what to choose when eating out at a Chinese restaurant:

- Steer clear of calorific starters. Spring rolls, prawn toast, crispy seaweed (which is, in fact, shredded cabbage and oil) are all high in fat.

▶

- Opt for soup as a starter. Chinese soups are often low in fat (containing about 3g per large serving).

- Ask for stir-fried vegetables instead of rice or noodles. If you do have rice, make it plain – a portion of boiled rice contains just 370 calories, whereas egg fried rice adds up to 625 calories and 32g of fat.

- Ask if the restaurant prepares its food with or without MSG. If possible, choose one that doesn't use this flavour enhancer (see page 245).

- Choose side orders of stir-fried vegetables or salad to fill you up.

- Avoid excessive salt, which means steering clear of the duck sauce, hot mustard, hoisin sauce and soy sauce.

- Leave off the sauce – it often adds the most calories in a dish.

- Eat with chopsticks – it can slow you down so that you eat less overall.

ADD UP THE EXTRAS

Calories can quickly add up when you're eating Chinese food. Keep tabs on what you are ordering by checking out the calorific values of the following:

Sesame prawn toasts: 70 calories each

Prawn wonton: 80 calories each   ➤

Crispy seaweed: 200 calories per portion

Spring roll: 165 calories

Prawn balls in sweet-and-sour sauce: 120 calories each ball

Spare rib: 145 calories each

Prawn crackers: 400 calories per bag

SWAP ▶ Crispy chilli beef

Per portion: calories 775; fat 31.1g; sugar 36g; salt 3.9g

Crispy battered, shredded or minced beef served with a hot dipping sauce was never going to be a low-calorie choice, given that it is deep-fried.

FOR ▶ Chicken chow mein

Per portion: calories 550; fat 19g; sugar 8.5g; salt 3.2g

Noodles, mushroom sauce, egg and chicken, plus vegetables, such as beansprouts and bamboo shoots, mean this is a better choice because you don't need to add rice or noodles – it's a meal in itself. It will save you over 200 calories. Swap the chicken for mushrooms and it boosts the vegetable content and lowers the calories by about 140; however, it also reduces the protein content of a meal, so serve alongside some other fish or meat dishes.

Fish and chips

Everyone knows that a fish and chip shop is hardly the place to visit if you are trying to lose weight, as almost everything on the menu is deep-fried. Nevertheless, they remain one of the most popular takeaway foods. Portion sizes are generally large, so savings can be made by sharing or asking for smaller servings. Avoid heaping on even more calories by adding extras like sauces and side dishes. There are some redeeming features to a fish and chip supper. For one, it is likely to contain no additives and flavourings, so you know what you are getting on that front. Fish contains protein and healthy fats. Trim off the batter (or ask for none) and you immediately shed a few hundred calories.

TOP SWAP TIP

Here's what to avoid and what to choose when buying from a fish and chip shop.

- The safest choice, while not exactly healthy, is a small cod and chips providing 838 calories and 48g of fat. It is still a high-fat meal and contains more than half the daily salt you need (3.1g), but it is a far better choice overall than, say, a beef and onion pie (which contains almost 500 calories) and plenty of stodgy carbohydrate in the pastry case.

- Opt for small or half portions of everything – chip shop sizes tend to be on the generous side. A large portion of battered cod and chips contains 1,385 calories and 77g of fat, a huge jump compared to the above.

- If you have a takeaway, tip the fish and chips onto kitchen paper before serving – it helps to absorb some of the excess fat.

- Avoid extras like white sliced bread, curry sauce or gravy, which can all add unnecessary salt.

▶

- Choose unbattered fish or chicken to save calories and fat. Some restaurants now serve grilled as an alternative. At the very least, discard the soggy batter that is right next to the fish.

- Select battered cod or haddock rather than plaice or rock, as they will save you calories. A small haddock contains 280 calories, a small battered cod contains 295, whereas a small battered plaice has 385 and rock 445.

- Swap chips for a portion of mushy peas or baked beans to go with your fish to save 700 calories and add protein.

- Swap a saveloy (235 calories) or sausage in batter (229) for a fishcake (186) to save on calories and fat.

It's not just the main meal that contributes to calories and fat. Be aware that added extras can send levels soaring.

ADD UP THE EXTRAS

Fish and chips represent a high-fat and high-calorie meal before you start adding extras. So be careful not to send levels soaring sky-high. Check out the values:

Pickled egg: 72 calories   Gravy: 98 calories

Mushy peas: 278 calories   Curry sauce: 130 calories

Pickled gherkin: 10 calories   Baked beans: 164 calories

Tartare sauce: *40 calories   Ketchup: *15 calories

*per sachet

Burgers

Once, burgers were considered the lowest of the low when it came to eating out and takeaways; they were so packed with fat and additives that they weren't to be touched with a barge pole. The rise of the gourmet burger bar has challenged that perception so radically that we now think of burgers as wholesome. Many fast-food outlets have also improved their offerings somewhat by cutting back on salt and frying using better quality oils.

Gourmet vs fast-food burgers

Does putting the word 'gourmet' in front of a burger and serving it in a stylish sit-down restaurant really make it that much better nutritionally than those dished out in, say, their fast-food rivals? The answer is a resounding no, at least when it comes to counting fat and calories, because the considerably more expensive burgers in many gourmet kitchens do no better than their supposedly downmarket rivals.

In fact, since gourmet burgers tend to be double the size of a fast-food burger, you can easily gobble double the calories in one sitting. Put this into context by considering that a cheeseburger from the Gourmet Burger Kitchen chain contains 805 calories and 55g of fat, almost twice as much as a McDonald's quarterpounder with cheese, which has 490 calories and 25g of fat. The gourmet version is much bigger and the size accounts for most of the differences, but add a side order of chips and you can see where things are heading.

How it's cooked counts

Serving sizes aside, there are advantages to going gourmet for your burger. Whereas most fast-food burger chains cook their meat on a steel griddle, where it sits in its own fat and absorbs some of it, the gourmet cooking method of choice is to chargrill, which allows the fat to drain away. The quality of ingredients used is generally better too, hence the higher price.

Hidden extras

About 15 additives are listed in the ingredients of many burgers sold in fast-food outlets, whereas gourmet burgers tend to contain very few, if any. In fast-food restaurants, burgers are usually frozen, and there have been concerns raised about the sources of the meat used.

A few years ago, a study in the *Proceedings of the National Academy of Sciences* journal made controversial claims about menu items served at fast-food burger outlets. Using a technique that identifies carbon and nitrogen isotopes in meat, the authors tried to determine the animals' diets and in what conditions they were raised. Based on the high levels of carbon and nitrogen isotopes found in the meat, they suggested the animals were predominantly fed corn, which makes them as fat as possible in as short a time as possible.

In the gourmet kitchens, burgers are freshly prepared using 100 per cent Aberdeen Angus beef sourced from traceable grass-fed cattle which, naturally, is far more reassuring partly because grass-fed cattle provide more monounsaturated fats. Furthermore, fewer artificial colourings and flavourings are found in the relishes and sauces used at upmarket burger bars, and they tend to contain less sugar, which is often added to disguise the flavour of additives in accompaniments at the cheaper end of the market.

Beware the obvious calorie pitfalls

There are nutritional howlers to be had in every burger establishment. The Smoked Bacon and Cheddar Double Angus burger at Burger King racks up a total of 966 calories and 58g of fat. Containing two 6.4oz burgers, bacon, Cheddar cheese, steakhouse sauce, lettuce, tomato, onion and mayonnaise, this monster burger is a recipe for disaster among dieters. Similarly, a gourmet burger with blue cheese and bacon can total almost 1,200 calories. For all-round quality of ingredients, the gourmet burger joints win hands down; just make sure you opt for smaller portions and skip the relishes, sauces and side orders.

TOP SWAP TIP

Here's what to avoid and what to choose at the burger bar:

- Avoid adding cheese and other toppings such as bacon and guacamole, which bump up the calories.

- Choose thick-cut chips over thin-cut fries, because a larger surface area means that they contain more potato and absorb less of the fat from frying.

- Fill up on extra veggies with your burger rather than relishes. Ask for extra tomatoes, onions and whatever other vegetables the restaurant offers.

▶

- If you have the option, always choose a wholemeal bun. Another great option is to go bunless, which saves you up to 200 calories. Gourmet bars often offer a choice of sourdough, which is a better option than plain white (see page 45).

- Don't be lured into buying a value meal, because it usually means adding a lot of unnecessary calories. Most value meals come with a medium order of fries, which adds about 290 calories.

Burger bars offer dozens of different toppings, relishes and sauces that can add up to an already calorie and fat-hefty meal. Be sure to choose wisely.

ADD UP THE EXTRAS

It's easy to add extras in a burger bar. Just be careful how many calories you are adding in the process. These values are per portion:

Hash browns: 390 calories	Ketchup: 20 calories
Regular fries: 290 calories	Onion rings: 398 calories
Large fries: 456 calories	Mayonnaise: *80 calories
BBQ dip: 50 calories	Slice of cheese: 75 calories

*per sachet

CHAPTER **TWELVE**

■

Drinks

Drinking eight glasses of water or healthy-sounding 'natural' drinks a day has long been considered the gospel of good living. Not only will it make your skin glow, we are told, but it will also help you to lose weight, flush toxins from your body and prevent headaches. What is less well known, however, is that these widely held beliefs were, in fact, largely dreamt up by bottled water manufacturers. In reality, they hold little water.

How much we actually need to drink on a daily basis has been at the centre of much scientific debate in recent years. What is now known is that there's little proof that drinking eight glasses or more of water a day wards off headaches or generally reduces appetite over the course of the day. And the belief that water boosts the excretion of toxins is not verified by any scientific study. The kidneys clear toxins independently of how much water you take in. Drinking lots of water to lose weight is also a waste of time. Even though some scientists have shown that women who drink water before or during a meal consume fewer calories at that sitting, researchers found no link between the amount of water 1,000 women drank and their weight or waist size.

Of course, water *is* required for all the body's cells to function and to excrete waste products, such as urea. And because we lose water all the time we do need to replace it by drinking fluids, but our bodies do a pretty good job of regulating water intake. When we need to replace fluids, our highly attuned accurate mechanism – good old thirst – kicks in, prompting us to take a drink. What's more, many foods that naturally contain large amounts of water – fresh fruit, vegetables, soups – contribute greatly to our fluid levels. Even tea and coffee, once considered the enemy of good hydration, are now known to help top up the body's water levels when consumed in moderation (four to six cups a day).

It's the type of fluid that counts

What we generally need less of, though, are so-called liquid calories: fluids that provide energy but don't leave us satiated. How the body regulates liquid calories from drinks is a hot topic of research. And it does seem that liquid sources of energy are handled in a different way from regular food by the body. Take fizzy or sparkling drinks. Researchers at Pennsylvania State University gave a group of adults an identical lunch on various days for six weeks and offered them a choice of either a regular or large sweet, fizzy drink, a diet fizzy drink or water before eating. When they took the large, sweetened fizzy drink, the subjects ate the same amount of lunch as on the days when they took water. In short, the sugary energy in the drink did nothing to stem their appetite or fill them up. In fact, since pre-meal water seems to stem appetite, it could be argued that the addition of sugar actually increases it.

Other studies have shown that similarly calorific fluids such as energy drinks, sports drinks and fruit juices have little effect on satiety. Although they add a sometimes significant number of calories, they don't result in you eating any less. What's more, many people underestimate the amount of sugar they consume in healthy-sounding drinks. In a survey by scientists at the University of Glasgow, it was found that pomegranate juice, for instance, contained 18 teaspoons more sugar than respondents thought.

How much fluid do we really need, and what type is best? The average man needs about 2 litres (3½ pints) daily and a woman needs 1.8 litres (3¼ pints) (more if it is hot or they are very active). Of the available drinks, plain water remains the best option and the only guaranteed calorie- and chemical-free beverage that is kind to the teeth as well as the waistline. It has also been shown to quench the thirst better than any other fluid.

WHEN LIQUIDS CAN AID WEIGHT LOSS

For many celebrities there is, it seems, only one way to lose weight, and that is to avoid food. Or at least to avoid chewing it. While diet fads that encourage the avoidance of a particular food group (carbs, fat, protein) come and go, there is one steadfast route to weight loss that appears to supersede trends: the liquid approach. From the maple syrup diet that requires followers to subsist on daily drinks alone, to the cabbage soup diet and the 'blend' trend for consuming puréed baby food, it's seemingly a case of swill (and then swallow) by mouth when it comes to achieving

▶

that A-lister form. Such approaches are far from healthy, since they advocate extremely low calories (and nutrients) and are simply unsustainable.

Emerging evidence does suggest, however, that there may be more benefits to consuming pulped and liquidised meals than was previously thought. There is no doubt that we have a physiological need to chew food and that the act of masticating helps to release and assimilate molecules of nutrients from food. It is thought that the longer a food remains in the mouth, as it does with solids, the more adept our tongues become at recognising its flavours, eventually sending messages to the brain to release the necessary digestive juices. Chewing and digesting food fills you up.

Yet, in one study, when dieters added puréed vegetables to some of their favourite dishes it helped them to shed pounds more quickly. Researchers gave 20 men and 21 women dishes such as casserole or macaroni cheese to which puréed cauliflower, butternut squash or carrots had been secretly added. While the subjects noted no changes in flavour, results showed they ate 200–350 fewer calories per meal when served the meals containing puréed vegetables. People who consumed a bowl of soup before a main meal reduced their overall energy intake by 20 per cent.

Although the ingredients remained the same – chicken stock, broccoli, potato, cauliflower, carrots and butter – the 'form' of the soups changed with those tested, including 'thin' broth, chunky vegetable soup and a fully puréed variety. Yet no matter how thoroughly it was blended, the soup was filling and helped dieters eat less. It is an area of

▶

research that is now intriguing nutritionists and scientists, but there can be little harm in filling up on nutrient-packed fluids such as healthy soups rather than empty calories and sugar in drinks.

Water

It is hard to imagine a time when water came mainly out of a tap. In the last thirty years bottled water has transformed itself from a rarity to the nutritional accessory of our time with the market currently worth over £2 billion a year. Few of us would be caught without a bottle of H_2O in our handbag, even though it costs 500 times more than tap water.

Do we know what we are drinking? Clever marketing campaigns mean that many consumers think bottled waters are a healthier choice. Yet there's little difference between tap and bottled water on a nutritional basis. Yes, mineral waters contain minerals, but in small amounts, and most of the minerals we need are obtained from food. The most important job of water is to keep people hydrated, and tap water does that as well as any. Here's a guide to water:

Tap water

All tap water is rain or melted snow collected from rivers, reservoirs and boreholes and treated before storage. Tap water is made 'safe' by various cleaning processes to neutralise it, then disinfected with chlorine. It sometimes has fluoride added. Leave tap water to stand for a few minutes before drinking it and the chlorine will evaporate.

It is now known that children are risking tooth decay as a result of drinking too much bottled water in place of tap water – a lack of fluoride in bottled water being to blame. Indeed, one study found that children who drank from 25 popular brands of bottled water had fluoride levels 26–48 per cent lower than those who drank fluoridated tap water.

DID YOU KNOW?

Water with a pH of more than 7.0 (which means it is alkaline) is generally recommended, because human blood is in the narrow range of 7.30 to 7.45 pH so it is more easily assimilated by the body than sugary drinks.

Spring water

EU regulations declare that spring waters must come from an underground source, be bottled under strictly regulated conditions and be microbiologically safe without treatment (although some substances such as iron and sulphur can be filtered out). No therapeutic claims can be made for spring waters. Taste-wise, there is little difference between spring water, mineral or tap.

Mineral water

According to EU directives, a natural mineral water must come from a single, identified source whose mineral salt content gives it specific properties that may be beneficial to health.

Any water that contains an appreciable quantity of dissolved minerals is described as 'hard water'. There are reputed health benefits to drinking hard waters regularly.

Naturally carbonated

This term means that the water emerges from underground with enough natural carbon dioxide to make it bubbly. According to EU regulations, the gas may be drawn off initially and then re-injected into the water on the bottling line. If a water is described as 'sparkling' or 'carbonated', it indicates the addition of artificial carbonation during the manufacturing process.

Table water

Table water (served in a bottle) can quite legally be sourced from a tap, and the contents are likely to be pretty much the same. It's no better (or worse) than tap water, so why pay about 28 times more for the privilege of putting it in a bottle?

Functional water

Did you think water was just there to hydrate? Not any longer. A virtual ocean of so-called 'functional' water drinks containing enhancements as diverse as ginseng, vitamins, bone-boosters and appetite suppressants are whetting the appetite so well that a report by market research analysts showed that they were the fastest growing sector of the soft drinks market.

As healthy as they sound, though, these functional drinks are not necessarily a welcome addition to the diet. Some of the drinks contain hidden sugars, with some having more calories per serving (about 120) than lemonade. Others are sweetened with fruit juice, which bumps up the calorie content; meaning that if you sip them as regularly as you might sip water it could lead to weight gain. In many cases the perceived benefits of vitamins in soft drinks are deceiving and the products are little more than a gimmick.

Are the added vitamins really worth it?

Unlike vitamin pills that contain nutrients designed to survive transit to the gut, those added to drinks are less stable. The shelf life and stability of vitamins is low and water-soluble vitamins – the B group and vitamin C – will break down over time, particularly if they are not refrigerated. By the time you finally consume a drink months after it was made it may well have lower amounts of nutrients than are listed on the label.

Beware of claims, too, that drinks containing ingredients such as B vitamins will provide an energy boost. They have little scientific basis. Most people get all the B vitamins they need from their diet, and even the weary can't expect a jolt from consuming extra in any form. So what should you swap? The values on the following pages are per bottle or serving.

DID YOU KNOW?

People with heart conditions are advised to check the labels of bottled waters for high levels of sodium. People with high blood pressure or who have had a stroke should check labels carefully and avoid products that contribute too highly to the recommended maximum of 2–2.4g of sodium a day for adults.

SWAP ▶ SoBe V Water Shield lemon and lime

Per 500ml (18fl oz) bottle: calories 85; fat 0g; sugars 18.5g; salt trace

V stands for vitamins and minerals. This drink has added potassium, calcium, magnesium, 25 per cent of the RDA for zinc and 200 per cent of the RDA for vitamin C, which are all reputed to boost the immune system. Although containing fewer calories per bottle than some functional drinks, this still has more than many cordials and squash drinks without significant nutritional benefits. There is no scientific evidence that the immune system would be boosted with such small quantities of vitamins.

FOR ▶ Bio Synergy skinny water

Per 500ml (18fl oz) bottle: calories 2; fat 0g; sugars trace; salt trace

The claims that Bio Synergy skinny water will help suppress your appetite and increase metabolism are linked to the added L-carnitine and chromium the drink contains. Both of these are natural substances that have been shown in some studies to minimise sugar cravings and to help burn fat more efficiently. Although it is true that L-carnitine and chromium have been linked to weight loss in some studies, the evidence is inconclusive and a lot of the research has been carried out on people who also exercise a lot. These drinks are not magic bullets for weight loss and the only guarantee you get with this swap is that you'll consume fewer calories than opting for a sugary-sweet, fizzy drink.

————

SWAP ▶ Glaceau Power-C vitamin water

Per 500ml (18fl oz) serving: calories 95; fat 0g; sugar 23g;
salt trace

This drink contains 200 per cent of our daily vitamin C and a
quarter of the necessary B vitamins and zinc. However, it also
contains added HFCS and sugar.

FOR ▶ Boot's Shapers sparkling lemon and lime

Per 330ml (11½fl oz) serving: calories 2; fat 0g; sugars trace;
salt trace

A carbonated spring water drink with natural flavourings,
preservatives and added vitamins and minerals. It is artificially
sweetened with sucralose. Other than being lower in calories
than the vitamin drink, it has no advantages on a nutritional
level, but it will save you 93 calories a drink.

Fruit and vegetable juices

In the last thirty years, fruit juices and, to a lesser extent, vegetable juices have become an accepted part of a healthy lifestyle. We guzzle them in the belief that their health-boosting
properties will improve everything from our complexion to
our lifespan, but there is more to many juices than meets the
eye. I know a lot of people who rather smugly sip several fruit
juices a day, thinking that they are nutritionally superior to
their coffee- or fizzy-drinking counterparts by filling their
bodies with freshly squeezed vitamins and minerals.

The concentrated sugars in fruit juices

What few juiceaholics realise is that although many of the colourful drinks may be full of nutrients they are also more sugary than fizzy drinks. Cola contains 26.5g of sugar, or just over five teaspoons, per 250ml (9fl oz) serving – less than many popular and exotic fruit juice products. And the sugar in fruit juice-based drinks can hold problems of its own. Although whole fruits are high in naturally occurring 'intrinsic' sugars, which are locked within the cells of a fruit, once a fruit is squeezed and juiced, its natural, healthy sugars are released to become partly 'extrinsic' sugars, which are known to promote tooth decay.

In fact, these sugars, combined with the acidity of many fruits, mean that a juice habit has been branded a potential dental disaster by some dentists. Every time you drink something acidic the enamel on your teeth is temporarily softened and loosened, and this can be very damaging. Sipping a juice over a prolonged period will extend the time your teeth are exposed to these acids, so it's best to drink a juice in one go. In the US, parents are urged to restrict their children's juice intake to one small glass a day by the American Academy of Paediatrics, who are concerned that, in addition to juices damaging dental health, too many fruit juices or smoothies are supplying 'liquid calories' that are fuelling the weight problems among pre-school children. Like other forms of sugar, fruit juices cause a sharp rise in blood sugar, triggering the body to store the resulting excess glucose as fat.

Drink fruit juices in moderation – once a day – and there are benefits. All fruit juices count towards one (but no more than one) of your recommended five-a-day servings of fruit and vegetables. Some provide a little fibre and many provide important amounts of vitamin C and minerals such as potassium.

Vegetable juices can be a better option as they generally contain less sugar, but they are still not a complete meal. Most vegetables can be juiced, but those with a high water content – tomatoes, cucumber, beetroot, carrots and lettuce – make a good base. Add broccoli, cauliflower, kale, spinach and celery for a real mix of flavours.

Home-juiced is best

Best of all are those fruit or vegetable juices that you juice or squeeze yourself. Not only are you guaranteed freshness but you can also select a variety of fruits or vegetables that provide a wide range of nutrients. If you are short of time or inclination, though, check which ready-made juices are the best on offer and which would be better swapped.

SWAP ▶ Cranberry juice

Per 250ml (9fl oz) serving: calories 135; fat trace; sugar 32g; salt trace

Contrary to popular belief, cranberry juice is not always useful for treating urinary infections such as cystitis, as studies have been unable to prove that even the fresh fruit is effective in combating the problem. Added to that, most cranberry juices are high in sugars and some of the more popular varieties are, in fact, sweetened with HFCS as well as sugar, which can combine to encourage bacteria to multiply, making cystitis worse. People with cystitis should avoid sugar as much as possible, including sugar in sweetened juices. If you want the benefits of cranberries, opt for the fruit itself.

FOR ▶ Non-smooth orange juice

Per 250ml (9fl oz) serving: calories 122; fat trace; sugar 25g; salt trace

Orange juice contains an antioxidant called hesperidin, which improves blood vessel function, helping to cut your risk of heart disease, as explained on page 127. A 250ml (9fl oz) glass such as this contains a full day's supply of immune-boosting vitamin C and 26 per cent of the RDA of folic acid. Because folic acid can't be stored by the body it needs to be supplied in food; it is important for a range of conditions including heart protection and the prevention of neural defects in unborn babies. In regular, smooth orange juice, the juicing process removes most of the fibre, but here a 250ml (9fl oz) glass will also provide you with just over 1g of fibre from the small pieces of orange it contains. It also saves a few calories and 7g of sugar per 250ml (9fl oz) compared to the cranberry juice.

SWAP ▶ Tropical fruit juice

Per 250ml (9fl oz) serving: calories 132; fat trace; sugar 34g; salt trace

This contains a mixture of juices including 45 per cent grape, 25 per cent orange and pineapple, mango and passionfruit juice. Bromelain, an enzyme in pineapple, is said to aid digestion and also to act as an inflammatory agent, easing the pain of aching joints, although more research is needed before the evidence is considered conclusive. There is no added sugar, but the sugars from the juices mean there is a lot per 250ml (9fl oz) and it will raise the risk of dental erosion if drunk too often, so limit to no more than a glass a day.

FOR ▶ Apple and pear juice

Per 250ml (9fl oz) serving: calories 115; fat trace; sugar 28g; salt trace

Drinking apple juice maintains your levels of a brain chemical called acetylcholine, which is vital for memory and brain health (low levels are linked to Alzheimer's disease), according to a US study. Thanks to its relatively high fibre content, it also aids digestion. A regular intake of pears has been shown to reduce the risks of strokes in susceptible people. But, bear in mind, that a whole apple contains 1.8g of fibre, whereas a 250ml (9fl oz) glass of this juice contains hardly any. Still, this is a worthy swap for the tropical fruit juice with fewer calories and less sugar per glass.

SWAP ▶ Apple and blueberry juice

Per 250ml (9fl oz) serving: calories 110; fat trace; sugar 26g; salt trace

A small study at the University of Cincinnati looked at the effect of blueberry juice on memory in adults in their seventies who had age-related memory decline. Those who drank a pint of blueberry juice daily for 12 weeks performed significantly better in memory tests. The problem with a drink like this is that it contains only around 1 per cent blueberry fruit juice, so you would have to drink a lot to make a difference to your health and that would mean plenty of extra calories.

FOR ▶ PomeGreat beetroot blend

Per 250ml (9fl oz) serving: calories 85; fat trace; sugar 20g; salt trace

Research at Queen Margaret University, Edinburgh found that drinking pomegranate juice causes a measurable drop in stress hormone levels. It can also help to lower 'bad' LDL cholesterol; research has shown that antioxidants in pomegranate juice may help to reduce the formation of fatty deposits on artery walls. Beetroot juice has been linked to lower blood pressure and also enhanced endurance in exercisers. This drink is relatively low in sugar, but it is made from concentrate that is reconstituted with water. Picking the seeds out of a fresh pomegranate and eating the fruit fresh is more therapeutic for your stress and nutrition levels than drinking the juice of the fruit. But the drink does save you 25 calories per 250ml (9fl oz) compared with the apple and blueberry drink.

SWAP ▶ AS10 superjuice

Per 250ml (9fl oz) serving: calories 170; fat trace; sugar 39g; salt trace

This 'super-drink' was commissioned by NASA after a study at the University of Pittsburgh revealed that the formula increased the lifespan of laboratory animals that had been given a lethal dose of radiation because of its very high antioxidant content. It contains no preservatives so, once opened, it can be stored in the fridge for no longer than two weeks. But it contains more sugar per glass than many juices. And it's worth pointing out that lab tests for the drink were performed on animals and such studies don't always reflect what happens once inside the human body.

FOR ▶ Strawberry juice

Per 250ml (9fl oz) serving: calories 110; fat trace; sugar 25g; salt trace

Strawberries are naturally packed with vitamin C – one serving of the juice contains more of the vitamin than an orange. They are also high in disease-fighting antioxidants known as polyphenols and have been shown in studies to boost brain power, lower blood pressure and protect the heart. Most strawberry juices are pasteurised, which means it can be kept un-chilled until opened, but it also means that many of the nutrients will have been destroyed during manufacturing. Better to juice your own. It does save you 60 calories and 14g of sugar per glass, however.

―――――――――

SWAP ▶ Welch's purple grape

Per 250ml (9fl oz) serving: calories 170; fat trace; sugar 41.25g; salt trace

This purple grape juice is made from the whole fruit, including the seeds and skin, of a variety of grapes known as Concord, which are native to North America. It carries Heart UK approval for a heart-healthy drink. The purple grapes have one of the highest levels of polyphenols (similar to that contained in Beaujolais red wine), which are thought to contribute to a healthy heart. In a study at the University of Cincinnati, psychiatrists found that a daily drink of grape juice improved patients' memory significantly compared with a placebo. Although it's good for the heart, it is among the highest in sugar content of all juices with over 8.5 teaspoons per 250ml (9fl oz), so if you want to drink it, it should be drunk sparingly.

FOR ▸ Sunsweet Californian prune

Per 250ml (9fl oz) serving: calories 162; fat trace; sugar 21.25g; salt trace

Prune juice is high in fibre and renowned for its ability to ease constipation gently and to aid digestion. A study at Florida State University showed that the fruit and juice helped prevent bone breakdown and osteoporosis in a group of postmenopausal women. Prunes are naturally sweet, but not excessively so and they also provide potassium, which can help to blunt the effects of sodium on blood pressure. A much underrated fruit and juice that will save calories and offer a health boost as well.

Smoothies

Fresh fruit crushed and pressed into a delicious smoothie seems like the ultimate health shot. In the UK, more than 30 million litres (6.5 million gallons) of smoothies are sold every year – an increase of 523 per cent since 1995. And those who drink them do so feeling virtuous about the vitamins, minerals and fibre they assume they're getting in every glass or bottle. For a nation that persistently fails to meet the recommended intake of five fruit and vegetables a day – most of us manage a paltry three – our appetite for these fruity drinks is surely good news.

Were you to make your own puréed and pulped drinks, the emerging evidence suggests that these liquid additions to the diet may indeed boost health and aid weight loss (see When Liquids Can Aid Weight Loss, page 258). But, on the commercial front there is no legal definition of the word 'smoothie', so any drink, regardless of how much (or how little) fruit it contains can currently claim to be one. To add to the confusion, manu-facturers often make misleading claims about the nutritional contributions smoothies make to the diet. Concerns have been raised because many commercially produced smoothies comprise mostly fruit that has been juiced with its fibre, skin and pith removed. Apart from the loss of healthy fibre, these important components of a fruit carry valuable nutrients, phytochemicals (which are beneficial plant compounds). Look out, too, for sugar, water and preservatives that are often added to the drink, which makes them little better than cola or lemonade.

Apple juice – a frequent bulking agent

A survey by Which?, the consumer watchdog, accused some manufacturers of misleading consumers by bulking up fruit smoothies with cheap apple juice and failing to mention this fact on the main product label. EU labelling laws are set to change, so that a smoothie can't be called 'strawberry and banana' when it contains 50 per cent apple juice, but in the meantime it's a good idea to read the ingredients' label just to make sure.

Smoothies at the premium end of the spectrum are a different story as many contain high levels of whole crushed or pressed fresh fruit and nothing else. As a guide, a top-end smoothie contains at least 80g (3oz) of fresh fruit per 250ml (9fl oz) serving, and provides 4.3g of beneficial fibre in the diet, representing 17 per cent of the GDA. Try the swaps below.

SWAP ▶ Asda pineapple, banana and coconut smoothie

Per 250ml (9fl oz) serving: calories 178; fat 2.75g; sugars 30.8g; salt trace

Fresh pineapple juice forms 39 per cent of the content and banana purée 36 per cent. But almost one-fifth of the drink's content is apple and orange juice. This is high in calories due to the coconut milk, the fat in which is mainly saturated. It's also among the highest in sugar content of commercial smoothies with sugars making up 12 per cent of its weight.

FOR ▸ Tesco mango and passionfruit smoothie

Per 250ml (9fl oz) serving: calories 150; fat 0.25g; sugars 32g; salt trace

Despite its name, the predominant ingredient is apple juice, comprising 47 per cent of this smoothie. A further one-fifth of its content is banana purée and orange juice, neither of which you would expect given the drink's title. Its sweetness is natural (from the fruit), though, and it saves you 28 calories per glass.

———

SWAP ▸ Sainsbury's berries and banana smoothie

Per 250ml (9fl oz) serving: calories 135; fat 0.25g; sugars 29g; salt trace

You wouldn't guess it from the title, but more than two-thirds of this smoothie is apple juice (52 per cent) and orange juice (17 per cent). In fact, banana and strawberry purées make up less than one-quarter of the drink's volume.

FOR ▸ Naked antioxidant mango juice smoothie

Per 250ml (9fl oz) serving: calories 130; fat 0.25g; sugars 29g; salt trace

The label boasts that there is 'a pound of fruit in every bottle', although the predominant ingredient is not mango, as you might expect, but apple juice. It provides a useful amount of fibre with 1.9g per 100ml (3½fl oz). Served in a tumbler, you would save a few calories, but be careful of the bottle size – a 450ml (16fl oz) serving is almost double the calories of a normal glass.

SWAP ▶ Sainsbury's vanilla bean and honey yoghurt smoothie

Per 250ml (9fl oz) serving: calories 280; fat 7.25g; sugars 40.25g; salt trace

This kind of smoothie takes the meaning of the term to a different level. Its main ingredient is whole milk yoghurt (71 per cent), but apple juice is the second highest on the ingredients' list. It is highly sweetened with 11 per cent honey and only a very small amount of vanilla beans for flavour. It provides more than one-tenth of a woman's recommended energy intake (2,000 calories) in a serving.

FOR ▶ Innocent strawberries and banana smoothie

Per 250ml (9fl oz) serving: calories 135; fat 0.5g; sugars 26g; salt trace

Although it does contain some apple, grape and orange juice, half this drink comprises the fruits it lists on the labels: 25 per cent whole, crushed strawberries and 25 per cent puréed bananas. Each 250ml (9fl oz) bottle or glass gives 135 calories and a useful serving of fibre (1g – 10 per cent of the GDA for an adult). It is unsweetened and all the sugars come from those in the fruit. Plus you slash the calorie count in half if you swap to this drink from the yoghurt smoothie.

SWAP ▶ Frobisher's orange, mango and banana smoothie

Per 250ml (9fl oz) serving: calories 56; fat 0.2g; sugars 10.4g; salt 0g

Positioned at the high end of the smoothie market (it is the only one tested that was packaged in a glass bottle), this Frobisher's smoothie contains fruit that has been pasteurised to prolong its shelf life. Despite its name, this one contains more apple juice than anything else (39 per cent) with banana and mango purées making up less than one-third of the product.

FOR ▶ Ella's Kitchen 'the red one' smoothie

Per 90g (3¼oz) serving: calories 47; fat 0.1g; sugars 10.4g; salt trace

A non-chilled, pasteurised product made from organic fruit. More than two-thirds of the content is bananas and strawberries, but one-quarter is apple juice. This product is actually marketed at children but, considering each tiny 90g (3¼oz) pouch provides almost one-quarter of a child's GDA for sugars, they would be much better off eating a banana and an apple. Still, for adults, you shave off a few calories per glass compared to the Frobisher's variety.

MAKE YOUR OWN

By far the best approach is to make your own smoothie. With a food blender or smoothie maker you can ensure that you add the entire fruit or vegetable, as well as varying

▶

the combinations and, therefore, the nutrients. Vegetables are generally a better smoothie ingredient as they have less sugar. If you do use just fruit, a cocktail of different varieties holds the most benefits. Scientists at the University of Strasbourg put 13 exotic fruits – including lingonberry, acerola and American chokeberry – into a blender to create a 'super-smoothie' that was shown in tests to relax the heart artery walls of pigs that consumed it. The researchers suggested it would probably boost blood flow to the heart in humans in a similar way. The findings also showed that the drink's antioxidant content helped to mop up free radicals, which can damage DNA and cells. Even the UK Department of Health has changed its guidelines when it comes to the contribution smoothies can make to your diet, although it is not advocating that all food is mushed up. Previously, pulped drinks could count towards only one portion of the recommended five-a-day, but now, provided a smoothie contains at least 150ml (5fl oz/¼ pint) of 100 per cent fruit juice (no added sugar or dairy, as in some commercial varieties) and 80g of pulped fruit or vegetables, it is said to count as two servings.

Sports and energy drinks

Billed as the ultimate workout accessory, sports and energy drinks are sold as products that will enable you to exercise harder and for longer so that you tone up and lose weight more quickly. But do energy drinks really enhance your fitness and boost your output at the gym? Many are simply sugar and water, so drinking them means you'll actually have to train longer or harder to shift the calories that you take in from the drink itself. They have their uses in endurance exercise, but the body is able to store enough glycogen (the fuel for exercise) to sustain 60–90 minutes of physical activity before the need to top levels up with carbohydrate-based energy products kicks in. In many cases, they just provide unnecessary extra calories.

Sports drinks and the sedentary lifestyle

It is when and why we are guzzling these products that is causing increasing concern. In a report by Mintel, it was revealed that nearly three-quarters of 16 to 24-year-olds say they take sports and energy drinks regularly, but often just because they like the taste – not to fuel significant activity. Likewise, recent research conducted by the National Hydration Council (NHC) found that over 11 million adults, including a quarter of all men, are sipping sports drinks while sitting at their desk. With the sugars in some energy drinks providing up to 350 calories per bottle it's not difficult to see how this excess energy heads straight for the waistline.

Regular sports drinks typically provide between 80 and 140 calories per bottle. In most cases, manufacturers now produce low-calorie versions of sports drinks, but even some of those contain 50 calories a bottle, which can mount up if you consume one or more a day. These products are designed for active people undertaking regular exercise lasting for longer than 45 minutes, but clever marketing means that people now think the ingredients will combat everything from fatigue and work-induced stress to hangovers. The drinks' association with sport triggers the idea that the products are healthier than, say, a carbonated drink. Although, actually, in terms of the amount of sugar they contain there is little difference – don't be fooled.

See where you can swap to save. Values below are per 500ml (18fl oz) serving:

SWAP ▶ Lucozade sport orange drink

Per 500ml (18fl oz) serving: calories 140; fat 0g; sugar 17.5g; salt trace

This is an isotonic sports drink – meaning it contains tiny particles of carbohydrate (or sugars) in the same concentration as the body's own fluids, so that they are easily absorbed. In this case, the carbohydrate mixture is glucose syrup and maltodextrin. Caffeine has been scientifically proven to improve alertness, which is useful for some sports. But you'd need to run at a decent pace for 20 minutes to burn off the calories in this.

FOR ▶ Lucozade sport lite orange drink

Per 500ml (18fl oz) serving: calories 50; fat 0g; sugar 5g; salt trace

This drink contains 70 per cent less sugars than regular sports drinks. You can easily replace the carbohydrate, fluid and electrolytes after an hour-long workout by drinking water or diluted fruit juice (which contains potassium, a mineral that is lost when you sweat) and eating a balanced diet when you finish; however, this is a much better choice than a regular sports drink if weight loss is the goal of your exercise regime, and it saves 90 calories per bottle compared with the regular version.

DIY SPORTS DRINK

What you need from an energy drink is fluid, sugar and a small amount of sodium to enhance fluid absorption from the gut as well as replacing some of the salt losses in sweat. To make your own version that is far cheaper than the commercial variety, mix diluted orange squash (not the sugar-free type) with a pinch of salt. It can be stored in the fridge for a couple of days.

SWAP ▶ Powerade original berry tropical drink

Per 500ml (18fl oz) serving: calories 80g; fat 0g; sugar 20g; salt trace

A startlingly blue coloured, isotonic sports drink, the original berry tropical drink contains a good blend of carbohydrate and fluid that will do what it says and maintain hydration while increasing energy through glucose. A good choice for serious exercisers, but with 100 calories per bottle, you would regain a quarter of the calories used in a typical gym class.

FOR ▶ Powerade zero berry tropical drink

Per 500ml (18fl oz) serving: calories 5; fat 0g; sugar 0g; salt trace

One of a newer range of drinks designed to appeal to gym-goers who don't want the calories in regular sports drinks; however, don't expect much of an energy boost. Of all the sports drinks looked at, this is the closest to plain water and isn't much better than drinking dilute squash, although the electrolytes it contains do aid fluid absorption from the gut. Still, it saves you 75 calories and cuts 20g of sugar from the original version.

SWAP ▶ Tesco active electro-lite lemon and lime

Per 500ml (18fl oz) serving: calories 50; fat 0g; sugar 11.2g; salt trace

This drink contains B vitamins and selenium, which are supposed to give an energy spurt, although you'd get more of them in a bowl of cereal and fruit. It is sweetened with HFCS, which has no scientific backing in terms of providing a long-lasting burst of sustained energy.

FOR ▶ High5 energy zero drink

Per 500ml (18fl oz) serving: calories 7; fat 0g; sugar 0g; salt trace

This product comes in tablet form and needs to be mixed with water. The tablets are a good idea, because it's easier to be accurate with the measuring than if you use mix-it-yourself powdered drinks. It's really important to measure out the water accurately, as too little will alter the fluid balance and may cause gastrointestinal problems during exercise. A peer-reviewed study at the University of Glasgow showed that exercisers burned an average of 41 per cent more fat when they drank this product compared to those who drank a regular isotonic sports drink. And it saves you over 40 calories compared with the 'lite' Tesco version.

Energy shots

Among the newest arrivals to the soft drinks market are tiny energy shot bottles that promise a quick energy boost when you need an instant lift. Unlike the older-style energy drinks, which are loaded with sugar, many of these new energy shots are sugar-free, containing only a few calories, although they often have the same amount of caffeine in each serving.

Not all energy shots contain high amounts of caffeine, however, and they have other ingredients such as vitamins, honey and sugar, but some provide far more than an espresso. Although caffeine can provide a temporary lift, it's important to stress that it acts only as a mental stimulant. It has been shown in trials to improve reaction times and focus, but caffeine does not provide or make energy and does not add to the body's energy reserves. Moreover, any effects are short term, and a cup of coffee would do the job just as well.

DID YOU KNOW?

The Institute of Advanced Motorists (IAM) in the UK, an organisation offering advanced training for motorists, issued a warning about energy shots, which are widely sold in garage forecourts and newsagents and promoted as a cure for tiredness. Research suggests that they can lead to lapses in concentration behind the wheel. A study by the US National Safety Commission revealed that motorists suffered delays in their reaction times an hour after taking highly caffeinated energy shots and drinks. This is because the boost from caffeine temporarily masks the effects of fatigue but does not offer a solution to tiredness.

How to get a more natural boost

Energy drinks can be ridiculously expensive and there are equally effective (and much cheaper) ways to replace fluids by using store-cupboard ingredients, as has recently been studied by researchers. Remember that these drinks are not intended for the average gym user or anyone who is just taking regular basic exercise; they are really only necessary for high levels of exercise.

Cherry juice Runners who drank cherry juice twice a day for five days before a marathon were shown to recover much more quickly and experience less muscle soreness than those who didn't.

Coconut water Proponents claim the low-calorie clear liquid from inside a coconut contains everything found in commercial energy products, including: water for rehydration; carbohydrates for energy; and electrolytes to replace what's lost through sweat. However, there is little scientific research confirming its benefits.

Chocolate milk Low-fat milk's mix of high-quality protein and carbohydrates can help refuel exhausted muscles. Scientists showed that after 2–4 days of intense training, chocolate-milk drinkers had significantly lower levels of creatine kinaise – an indicator of temporary muscle damage – compared to those who took sports drinks.

Beetroot juice Drinking 500ml (18fl oz) of beetroot juice a day for a week helped sporty subjects to cycle 16 per cent longer before getting tired out. Drinking the juice doubles the amount of nitrate in the blood and reduces the rate at which muscles used adenosine triphosphate (ATP), their main source of energy.

Slush drink Drinking a slushy ice drink just before running on a treadmill in a hot room could keep you going for an average of 50 minutes before having to stop. It's thought that the crushed ice drink lowers body temperature, allowing runners to run for longer before their bodies became critically hot. It also appeared to prevent heart rates from soaring too quickly.

Flat cola Caffeine (from flat cola or cold black coffee) has become one of the most widely studied ergogenic aids in sport. Caffeine works by triggering the release of body fats into the bloodstream during activity. This means that fat is burned during exercise rather than carbohydrate, the body's primary choice of fuel, and endurance capacities are improved.

Alcoholic drinks

Dieters who religiously tot up the calories in the food they consume could undo their attempts at healthy eating by having an alcoholic drink with or after their meal. Surveys have shown that two out of three Britons are unaware of how many calories are contained in their favourite tipple; that bottle of wine you share at the weekend could contain the same amount as a New York cheesecake. UK guidelines recommend men drink no more than four units a day and women no more than three, with two alcohol-free days per week and no more than 21 units per week for men and 14 units per week for women.

SWAP ▸ Lager
Per pint: calories 233

FOR ▸ Guinness
Per pint: calories 210

———

SWAP ▸ Alcoholic ginger beer
Per bottle: calories 254

FOR ▶ Beer
Per pint: calories 182

————————

SWAP ▶ Champagne
Per 120ml glass: calories 91

OR

SWAP ▶ White wine
Per 125ml glass: calories 92

FOR ▶ Red wine
Per 125ml glass: calories 85

————————

SWAP ▶ Sherry
Per 50ml glass: calories 139

FOR ▶ Rosé wine
Per 125ml glass: calories 89

————————

SWAP ▶ Gin and tonic
Per single/small pub measure: calories 213

FOR ▶ Pimm's and lemonade
Per standard serving: calories 85

————————

SWAP ▶ Sex on the beach
Per standard serving: calories 150

FOR ▶ Bloody Mary
Per standard serving: calories 140

————————

SWAP ▶ Bellini
Per standard serving: calories 158

FOR ▶ Mai tai
Per standard serving: calories 125

SWAP ▸ Long Island iced tea
Per standard serving: calories 270

FOR ▸ White wine spritzer (with soda)
Per standard serving: calories 132

———————

SWAP ▸ Martini (vermouth)
Per standard serving: calories 99

FOR ▸ Vodka
Per single/small pub measure: calories 72

———————

SWAP ▸ Mojito
Per standard serving: calories 111

FOR ▸ Cosmopolitan
Per standard serving: calories 99

———————

SWAP ▸ Black Russian
Per standard serving: calories 125

FOR ▸ Bacardi and diet coke
Per single/small pub measure: calories 52

———————

SWAP ▸ Pina colada
Per standard serving: calories 280

FOR ▸ Baileys Irish cream
Per standard serving: calories 130

———————

SWAP ▸ Zombie
Per standard serving: calories 325

FOR ▸ Margarita
Per standard serving: calories 145

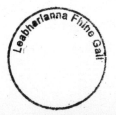

Index